Eat Ice Cream *for* supper

Kathy has written this book as an inspiration to others. She faced cancer twice, first with the diagnosis of her husband with rectal cancer, and then a few years later with her diagnosis of breast cancer. In this book, Kathy shares useful advice and words of comfort with her readers. Her book is a faith-based practical approach to coping with the diagnosis of cancer and loss. It is a realistic, heartfelt description of the cancer journey and the inspiration that can be found in the Bible.

—**Hilah Sue Perkins**, ARNP

Kathy's book, *Eat Ice Cream for Supper,* is one of the essential resources you need in your toolkit when fighting cancer or supporting someone through their journey!

—**Joy Huber**, Author of *Cancer with Joy,*
Stage 4 Young Adult Cancer Survivor,
Huffington Post Blogger & Professional Speaker

Eat Ice Cream
for supper

A Story of My life with Cancer
A GUIDE FOR YOUR JOURNEY

God is our refuge and strength,
a very present help in trouble.
Therefore will not we fear …
—Psalm 46:1–2

Kathy Manning Gronau

NEW YORK

Eat Ice Cream *for* supper
A Story of My life with Cancer.
A Guide for Your Journey

Published in New York, New York, by Morgan James Publishing. Morgan James and The Entrepreneurial Publisher are trademarks of Morgan James, LLC. www.MorganJamesPublishing.com

The Morgan James Speakers Group can bring authors to your live event. For more information or to book an event visit The Morgan James Speakers Group at www.TheMorganJamesSpeakersGroup.com.

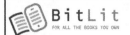

FREE eBook edition for your
existing eReader with purchase

PRINT NAME ABOVE

For more information,
instructions, restrictions, and
to register your copy, go to
www.bitlit.ca/readers/register
or use your QR Reader to scan
the barcode:

ISBN 978-1-61448-814-9 paperback
ISBN 978-1-61448-815-6 eBook
Library of Congress Control Number:
2013945994

Cover Design by:
Rachel Lopez
www.r2cdesign.com

Interior Design by:
Bonnie Bushman
bonnie@caboodlegraphics.com

In an effort to support local communities, raise awareness and funds, Morgan James Publishing donates a percentage of all book sales for the life of each book to Habitat for Humanity Peninsula and Greater Williamsburg.

Get involved today, visit
www.MorganJamesBuilds.com.

**Habitat
for Humanity®**
Peninsula and
Greater Williamsburg
Building Partner

Dedication

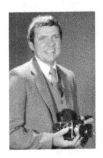

*This book is dedicated to
the memory and life of Orin P. Gronau
1945–2007*

Your Greatest Gift

Some men spend time on earth building great wealth, fame, knowledge, and degrees.

Not so was the man I married—when I was too young to even know the true gift that God had chosen for me. It was to be many years before I would have the wisdom to truly understand.

Orin was a man who took care of his home. He did what needed done. The filters got changed and the eaves troughs were cleaned. He always remembered. He was faithful.

Orin took care of his children. Their needs were met; they were loved. His children were the center of his world. Little league and pigeon shows were always more important than golfing or such. No need to buy a batting pole, daddy made one.

When his sons brought him new daughter-in-laws they were as his own, he helped them with whatever was needed. It was always the same, "the boys were busy and it needed done."

Orin loved his grandchildren; every one of them was precious to him. He loved them all and enjoyed them immensely. You didn't go to grandpa's without sharing his M&Ms—but you behaved—until almost the last day grandpa was known to say "KIDS, PICK THAT UP!"

Orin loved his wife: at fourteen he met her at the county fair, at sixteen he gave her an engagement ring, and at nineteen made her his bride. On August 25, 2007, we would have celebrated forty-two years of marriage. Some years were hard. Orin knew how to stay. He learned how to love, and he did it daily with his heart and his life, showing it as much in the things he did as the words he said. He always worried more about my needs than his. Even in his last days he would refuse to wake me in the night because I needed my sleep.

Orin was a faithful friend. When help was needed, help was given. It was how it was done and now I watch with pride as his sons do and give as they were taught.

Orin belonged to the Lord. When he decided to follow Christ, he loved Him like he had always known to love. He served as he had always served—with his heart and his hands. In the church building, examples of his work remind us: the welcome bench in the foyer, the sound equipment station, and a basement remodeled.

But the greatest gift is that of a gentle man who got it—who understood that LOVE was not a feeling but a DOING. Quietly, without asking for notice or praise, he exemplified what God's Word says in the book of James: a faith that works.

Thank you, Orin, for teaching me how to love. Your dearest wife,

Kathy

Table of Contents

Foreword

Cancer.

Few expressions in our language evoke a myriad of feelings as this one simple word. Panic, fear, anger, denial, unbelief—they go on and on. Few people in this world have not been touched by it, either directly or indirectly. Ultimately we will all have to ask, "What do we do now?" When confronted with this most ominous of words, we need to step back, get a grip on the vast scope of what is to come, and begin to walk forward. That is precisely what *Eat Ice Cream for Supper* can help you do.

It is poignant, it is practical, it will make you laugh, it will make you cry, but most of all, through the pages of this book you will find the courage and the know-how to go on.

—Karen Manning Wilson

Preface

I have a great family. I was raised in a two-parent farm home with two sisters. We attended church on Sunday, had chores, worked hard, and played paper dolls, cowboys and Indians, and chased fireflies on warm summer evenings. Mom, at ninety-five, remains the matriarch for us and our extended families. My two sons, Scott and Mike, and their wives have blessed us with five biological grandchildren and several more step grandchildren, all of whom bless my life.

We are a close family, so when cancer struck—not once but twice—first my husband and then me, it changed our plans, our dreams, and our lives, not only in our household, but in every one of the others. Those cancers, occurring in 2004 and 2007, were enclosed almost like parentheses by the sudden death of my father in 1996 and my nephew in 2013.

This is our experience. Written to be a guide through the medical process of diagnosis, treatment, and end of life, my desire is that it will give you comfort, a smile, information, and encouragement.

.

Acknowledgments

To my son Mike Gronau without whose tireless efforts and persistence this book might never have been completed, you are a joy to my heart.

To my son Scott Gronau who believed in me and provided quiet encouragement; and to my grandson Blake, who suggested I needed a German shepherd dog to protect me when I was a famous author, thank you for being there.

To my amazing daughter-in-law Emily, to Allison, and to my grandchildren who love me unconditionally and provide the *why* for all I do, thank you!

To my mother, Geneva Manning, who nursed me through chemo rounds, stood by my side through Orin's illness, and understands my widowhood like no one else. What a blessing you have been in all our lives.

To my sisters Karen Wilson and Rita Lyon who believed in my writing, took notes at oncology appointments, edited my manuscripts, and who still cook many great meals when I visit, you are just the best!

To my sister-in-law June Young who has become a dear friend and sister over the years, and who shares my hobbies, smiles, and tears; I don't even know how to begin to thank you for all you've done, but thank you.

To my niece Debbie Church who has always had time for her Uncle Orin and Aunt Kathy. Thank you for your love and caring, and for allowing me to use your stories in this book.

To Jenny Collins who always encouraged me and reminded me of God's purpose when I needed it most, you are an amazing friend.

To my pastor Mike Buckamneer and his wife Jane who have stood with me through the worst. God will surely have crowns waiting. Thank you for never giving up.

To my cousin Julane Hiebert who asked me to go with her to that first CWF meeting and who, along with Sara Meisinger and Susan Mires, prayed, prodded, and applauded the entire way. You are my heroes!

To critique partners, Joyce Love, Carol Russell, Sally Smith, Julianne Harlan, and Suzanne Cisco who spent tireless hours each week reading and correcting my manuscript, thank you all!

A very special thanks to Terry Whalin, acquisitions editor at Morgan James Publishing, who persisted in securing this book for publication; to editor Tanya Brockett of Hallagen Ink who worked to put the rough beginning into a polished, publishable document; and finally to Morgan James Publishing for consistent and quality work at every step. Thank you all.

May God bless you richly.

Introduction

There is a reason God gives us only one day at a time. Yesterday is too big a burden to carry and tomorrow too fearful to see.

This book is a product of a daily walk—one that included heartaches, laughter, loss, and recovery. It can be read all the way through or used as a reference with each chapter being complete in addressing a specific topic, including the following sections:

- Survival Tips—Things that you can do to cope and conquer.
- What a Friend Can Do to Help—How to be helpful when you don't know what to say or do.
- Points to Ponder—Thinking about the issues from a spiritual perspective.

··

Part One
Our Story

Every story has a beginning.
This is ours.
Life is hard.
So is staying.
Change happens.
Decisions aren't always the best ones.
God is still God.
Praise Him anyway.

··

Chapter One

In the Beginning

• •

"How was your day?" I asked.

"Not good," my husband replied. Then hesitating, he said the words that changed my world.

• •

I Had a Hero

I didn't just marry my sweetheart; I grew up with him. We met when I was thirteen and he fourteen.

It was the most romantic of spots! The sights and smells left no doubt as to the location. It was opening day at the County Fair. My 4-H steer was in the stall next to his.

For two years he courted me, first on Sunday afternoons and by mail, the old fashioned kind, with paper and ink and a four cent stamp. Finally, we were allowed to double-date with his sister and her fiancé.

At seventeen, he graduated from high school and joined the Air Force, giving me a diamond ring before he left.

At nineteen, I married him. He was my sweetheart, and I his. Stationed at the Air Force base in North Dakota, we skated and sledded in the wonderland winters. Two years later, in Kansas we started a business, had babies, fought a little, and loved a lot.

At sixty-one, the doctor had bad news. Together, as always, we fought the battle. He left me one night, when the battle was over; flew off with the angels, his pain finally gone. I looked at my boys, there beside me, and remember telling them to love their wives like their dad had loved me. It hadn't always been easy. We had our share of problems. But he always stayed. I was who I was because of him. He had given enough.

His love still sustains me. On quiet nights I remember the County Fair, and its sights and its sounds and its smells …

Storms

After thirty-nine years of marriage with all its ups and downs, my husband and I had finally accepted and made firm commitments to serve the Lord and each other. Life was good. For the first time in many years we again worked together and enjoyed our shared lives on the job and at home. Our children were happy; our four-year-old grandson was our pride and joy. Our first granddaughter was on the way. Though we had suffered minor health issues, we were blessed with better than average health, and looked forward to years of fun and service in our retirement years. We had carried through with regular yearly physicals, but one test had been ignored. Ignored. Avoided. Forgotten.

It can take ten years for a polyp to turn into a cancerous tumor.

At sixty-one, my husband was eleven years overdue for a first screening colonoscopy. Vague symptoms, not well followed or explored were blamed on arthritis from bouncing along in an eighteen-wheeler.

And then there was the day when the bleeding signaled the alarm.

Rectal bleeding is one of those things that everyone hates to talk about. It's embarrassing. It's alarming. It's a signal something is wrong. *It might be a simple hemorrhoid. But it might be so much more.* Questioning, I believed the first. *Bright red blood,* I thought, *that's good.* He had told me days earlier that he was having trouble. I mistakenly thought he was describing constipation. *That would explain the bleeding.*

Then he said the words that changed my world—"I'm having trouble going—it's like a pencil when it comes out."

A lecture from a long ago class in nursing school flashed in my head. I remembered those symptoms as signaling an obstruction in the colon. My heart sank and my mind whirled as the meaning of the two symptoms gelled.

"You need to see the doctor; tomorrow. Shall I call or will you?"

So began our journey. Our town is small and our doctor an old friend. The call indeed resulted in an appointment that very next day, followed by a referral and appointment with the surgeon. The colonoscopy was scheduled within the week.

Another Beginning

It was six o'clock in the morning as we drove out of the driveway. I wondered if my life would ever be the same again. That was the beginning. And it was also the end. The end of what seemed to me had only begun. I was no longer a teenage bride, bright with anticipation of a whole lifetime ahead. I was no longer part of mom and dad, no longer even part of the *us* who had matured into the quiet life of middle age; all of it seemed to vaporize with one word, cancer. I had known even before the doctor told me—known with the admission by my beloved only days before, of medical problems and symptoms and meanings and outcomes. Somehow, I knew.

My first reaction was to cry, "Not me, not him." Instead, as a nurse, I slipped into the caregiver role I was taught. I knew what lay ahead. Even now, years later, I feel and remember the adrenaline that pushed me into that role. In it I could be strong and competent; I would face and deal and conquer.

There would be times of doubt, but I believed God. I knew He would not let us down, whatever came to pass.

Looking back, I have few regrets. He became my priority. His care mattered most. All else came second. Only one thing was as important and on that we agreed. I would continue to take our grandchildren to Sunday school and church each Sunday. When he could go we rejoiced. When his illness made it impossible, we rejoiced that I could get them there. He would wait on those days for my return and the report of how the morning had gone.

It is easy to look back and see what you should have done. It is worthless ruminating; worthless, that is, unless it helps someone else. After seeing what his dad went through, one of my sons started having a colonoscopy at forty, knowing this was a small inconvenience that would have saved his dad's life. In fact, colonoscopies are no longer too much trouble in our extended family either. More than one family member, following up on the admonition to have the procedure, reported polyps removed—cancer prevented.

In the third year of my husbands' cancer treatment, the AFLAC representative showed up at my workplace. Realizing how expensive treatment had been, even with good insurance, I knew we would never financially survive if I got sick also.

The agent did the figures for me: if my husband had owned the policy, it would have paid us about $30,000 at that point; money that could have paid deductibles, the house payment, gas, lodging, and food expenses. I was convinced. I took out a cancer policy. One year later, having the policy helped me as a widow to survive my own bout with cancer treatment and its expenses. Specialized policies are available for not just cancer, but for other things such as stroke or heart attack. Especially if you have a strong family history of such illnesses, it might be well to consider including one in your financial planning.

Survival Tips

- Listen when your loved one has unusual complaints. Don't ignore them. Don't let the doctor ignore them either.

- Know your family history; it can be a powerful tool.
- Buy cancer insurance BEFORE you go to the doctor.
- Pray. Hebrews 4:11 tells us we "can come boldly to the throne of grace." Now is the time to go. Go for your loved one, go for the doctors you will see, and go for yourself.
- Be patient. Tests take time. So does waiting. Allow it. Know that God has it all figured out even when you don't.
- Be kind. Anxiety can cause us to be short-tempered, impatient, and demanding. Resist.

What a Friend Can Do to Help

- Be there. Our pastor was rather new to our church and we were barely more than acquaintances. It was a colonoscopy. Not a procedure that would normally require a pastor's presence. Yet he was there. He said little that was of importance. I only know that when the surgeon came out and said, "There's a little room over here where we can talk," my pastor waited with me, and prayed with me, and said little else, but he was there.
- Listen. So many things are probably going on inside your loved one's head right now. What they need most is just a place to voice them. You don't have to have the answers. In fact, it is better if you don't. They don't need answers anyway, at least not from you. They do need to know they aren't alone.
- Don't give pat answers or trite reassurances. It was far more reassuring to me to hear that someone had heard the worst and survived than to be told, "don't worry, I am sure it will be okay."
- Encourage evaluation. It is so easy to slip into "it will never happen to me" thinking. If your friend does that, gently, but firmly, guide them back into moving forward.
- Pray. Pray now for your loved ones and for the doctors. Pray for calmness, for wisdom, for the ability to hear, for faith, and for mercy.

Points to Ponder

> *Be not afraid of sudden fear, neither of the desolation of the wicked, when it cometh. For the LORD shall be thy confidence, and shall keep thy foot from being taken.*
> **—Proverbs 3:25–26**

I love it when the Word of God is so clear on an issue that you don't even have to pray about it! This verse is one of those. Sudden fear happens to us frequently. It's the dread when the phone rings late at night. It's the feeling of helplessness as you lay on the exam table, waiting while the doctor examines the lump that you found. It is screeching tires or the realization while shopping that your three-year-old is nowhere in sight. It's the concern for a loved one or friend that God gives you when He wants you to pray.

Sudden fear grips all of us at some time or another. Its power is in the fact that it is—well—sudden. God says, "Don't be afraid of that."

On first look, it seems as if this verse is saying that we shouldn't be afraid at those times when we are caught off guard by an event that might result in something bad. The Bible has in many places assured us that Jesus will not leave us; that the Holy Spirit is with always with us; that as a Christian we cannot be plucked from the Master's hand. We are to trust, lean, cleave, hide in, and be upheld.

This verse is different. In some places we are told not to fear trials, tribulation, even death. Here however, we are told not to be afraid of fear, or more specifically, sudden fear. I think God is reminding us that there are times when fear has a good and useful purpose in our lives, stopping us from doing things that would hurt, or preparing our hearts to handle difficult news. God seems to be saying, there are times when you need to be on your toes and now is one of them, don't be afraid of it, I am still here, but pay attention.

Sudden fear can paralyze if you allow Satan to trick you into thinking that something awful, disastrous, and uncontrollable is about to happen. It is easy to fall into the trap of not trusting God at a time when we most need to trust. Don't let that happen. The next time something causes "sudden fear," instead of running to hide, praise and thank Him for His warning that remembering to trust Him is never more important than right now. Pay attention. Stop before you fall in that hole again. Gather your young ones close. Change your course. Proceed with caution. Do all this, not trembling but boldly because God says, even in fear, I am. I AM.

Chapter Two

Dealing with the Diagnosis

. . . .

I watched as the surgeon came down the long
hall, and tried to read his thoughts, or interpret
his expression, and then felt dread reach out and
pull me in as he said, "There's a private room just
over here where we can talk."

. . . .

My Experience

Few words have the ability to get our complete attention while sending
us immediately into a state of dazed shock. Cancer is one of those words.
As I sat in that tiny office, my pastor at my side, I heard the word likely
to change my world forever. My husband had gone in for a colonoscopy
because of bleeding. I hoped for a diagnosis of hemorrhoids, and instead

I heard "tumor in the lower colon"—a tumor so big that the doctor would not send him home, instead recommending surgery immediately. Thus began a three-year journey into the unknown.

STOP

> **S—Stop:** Do not be pressured into a decision until you have the facts.
>
> **T—Talk:** Tell each other what you are thinking and feeling.
>
> **O—Options:** Remember, you have options.
>
> **P—Pray:** Pray and proceed with what you believe is the right thing.

My Reaction

Cancer treatment was a new and unfamiliar experience for me. I am a take charge, figure-out-what-to-do and "get it done" sort, and treating cancer is so much the opposite. Daily the scene changes on treatment options as new research and new drugs surface. Treatment recommendations in other fields of medicine are usually clear cut. There may be choices, but each choice is clearly defined, complete with benefits and risks. With cancer treatment, however, there are also often choices that can be made to try promising yet unproven treatment through clinical trials and frequent new medications and treatments being released. Never will you need the Lord's guidance as much as now. Before you do anything, stop. Stop. Pray. Learn. Knowledge is power. This is not the time to pretend nothing is happening. Much is. That <u>much</u> demands decisions you and your loved one will need to make. Some before you are ready. But STOP.

S—Stop. Don't be pressured into a decision until you have prayed and have all the facts.

When my husband's tumor was found, we were told and believed that surgery was the immediate need. When that was over, we were referred to an oncologist. The appointment was made. We went and there learned of and began treatment. In retrospect, it would have been good to have seen the oncologist prior to surgery. It would have been good to have been given a choice. It would have been good if we had had someone who would process with us what was happening and what was about to happen. That person is out there. Find them. Of course, don't wait weeks to begin, but a few days to seek advice and a second opinion not only make sense for you, but will ensure the best possible treatment in the end.

T—Talk. Tell each other what you are thinking and feeling.

Remember that in most cases the person with the diagnosis must make the treatment choices. You are there to listen, ask appropriate questions, and help digest and interpret the information.

O—Options. You have options.

There is always more than one way to address a problem and it's no different with medical issues. In fact, sometimes, cancer treatment is ALL about options; all about choices.

P—Pray. Pray and proceed with what you believe is the right thing.

My pastor (Mike Buckamneer, Pastor, Crossroads Baptist Church in Girard, Kansas) gives this advice. Keep reading your Bible every day. When you ask God to guide you, you do not have to go paging through the index to find the answer. He will show you. That day, that week, that month, when it is the right time for you to know, a verse will seem to pop off of the page. It may not have anything to do with your question directly, but somehow you will know. The verse, that day, that time, will mean something different to you than to possibly anyone else in the room. It will be just for you.

Your Loved One's Reaction

Understand that you and your loved one may be at different places emotionally with the diagnosis. It can be helpful to find someone who can just listen, without giving too much advice, while you sort out your thoughts, feelings, and fears.

Knowledge is your friend. Seek it.

Asking Questions

When it was my turn to be the patient, I wasn't always the nurse. I don't even remember the first time we saw the oncologist. When discussing this book with my son, he recalls that I appeared very anxious and stressed at that first appointment, wanting to take the most aggressive treatment route possible. Instead, he relates, the doctor was very calming in his approach, suggesting that I take a deep breath. I had just lost my husband and now the doctor who had been his primary oncologist was going to be my doctor. Having visited with me on numerous occasions when I accompanied Orin, the doctor realized I would compare my situation to that of my husband's and provided reassurance that this was a different situation with very likely a different outcome. When my husband was diagnosed several years earlier, we knew little and asked few good questions, most of which we thought of after we arrived for the appointment. Both of these are examples of why it is important to prepare for the appointment and take someone along.

Three years later, when I saw the specialist, I took my sisters to the appointment with me. They helped me listen and we had a full page of questions prepared. My sister kept notes and prompted me when I seemed not to be remembering what to ask.

It is not uncommon to jump to the end, so to speak, without reading the book. The doctor says cancer and we want to know if we are going to die. The answer to that is yes. Unless Jesus comes first, we will all one day, some way, die.

We want to know what, when, how, and probably why. The doctor does not have the answer. He might be able to predict based on the facts he has gathered up to that point, but it is really only a guess. God is the one who has those answers, and one day you will stand before His throne and you can ask.

So having said that, let's get good at finding out what will help you move forward. Some of those questions you do not need to ask your doctor or at least your doctor only. Still, they will most likely center around the what, when, how, and whys that I mentioned earlier.

The questions will likely depend also on whether you/your loved one are/is a feeler, thinker, or doer. You are likely wondering where this is going. Trust me. You may have the same questions, but how you process information will affect what and how you will ask.

Different People/Different Questions: o
Feelers—Thinkers—Doers

Feelers are people who need to feel good about the information or decision. Thinkers need to understand. They need the facts, need them in order, need them complete, and will ask three times as many questions in the process. Doers, just do. They don't need to feel good about it or understand it. It is important that you figure out your tendency, as you are called upon to take a greater role in the decision-making and care.

In our situation, I was and am a thinker. I am probably not going to buy in to anything that I don't understand. I need to somehow let the medical team in on this little secret. Orin, however, was a little bit feeler and a lot doer. I would struggle to figure it all out, get it in the right order, understand the pros and cons, etc. He would hear, accept, and act.

Look at some examples of questions and address them by these personality types. For example, *what*: What do I have, where did it come from, what is it called, etc.

- Doers likely want to know what they have, and then they will jump directly to what they need to do about it. Their questions look like this:

- o Do I have cancer?
- o Where is it?
- o Can I survive it?
- o What will my treatment be?
- o When do I start?
- o How long will it last?
- o Will I be sick?
- o Can I keep working?
- Thinkers will want to know all of the above, but they will also want to know:
  - o What kind of cancer is this?
  - o How do you diagnose it?
  - o What kind of research has been done in treating it?
  - o What are the survival statistics?
  - o When I come for treatment, where will it be? Who will do it? Are they experienced?
  - o How long will I be here for each treatment?
- Feelers will be more concerned with how it affects both them and you.
  - o Will the cancer make me sick?
  - o Will it hurt?
  - o Will the chemo treatment take a long time?
  - o When will I have treatment?
  - o What can I do? Is there a TV?
  - o Can I sleep if I want to?
  - o Should I bring lunch?
  - o Do you think I should do this?
  - o What will I do if I am scared, sick, and unable to care for myself?
  - o What do you think we should do?

A doer wants to know that someone is in charge and directing the show. If so, they will follow. A thinker's decision about the right medical team addresses knowledge and the ability to communicate. A feeler will make the decision on their medical team because "it feels right"—it is as much about the relationship as it is about the professional treatment. It may be the doctor who has a special way of showing that he really cares. It may be about the nurses who ask about your grandkids and listen to your fears. It may be about the office staff that light up when you arrive and you know it's not just a job to them.

The right treatment team will make the journey easier, even if it isn't pleasant. Usually it will be a combination of people who are different. You will likely find yourself migrating to the ones who communicate with your style. That's okay. It's one of the beauties of having multiple people on your treatment team.

See the *Appendix* for a suggested list of questions to ask your doctor.

Searching the Internet

There is so much information available on the web that it is almost a sin to remain ignorant about your condition. That said, however, it is absolutely necessary that you pay strict attention to who you are reading. There isn't an Internet police who stamps a big red warning sign on web addresses of biased or unreliable information.

Sometimes a quick look at the web address will give you a clue. If it is labeled something odd like MiracleCuresUsingOnlyChocolateMilk. com, that may be your first clue. (Although I have been known to think chocolate could cure quite a bit of things!)

Reliable sites are usually those that aren't selling something or promoting one person or group. I found information on the sites of National Cancer Centers, such as www.mayoclinic.com to be helpful. Government sites such as www.nih.gov and www.cancer.gov also offer a wealth of reliable information as well as links to other good sites.

Your Physician or Cancer Treatment Facility

Many physicians and hospitals have a wealth of information in the form of small pamphlets, booklets, and even CDs that they will give you. These can be great places to gain information without being overwhelmed by the vast amount found on the web.

Although I found most all of the professionals that I dealt with to be helpful, I found our nurse practitioner to be the very best one to go to when I didn't understand. She had the knowledge I needed and the skill to teach it.

I also recommend *Cancer with Joy*, a book with a wonderful list of websites and what they offer by Joy Huber. The book can be ordered from her website at www.cancerwithjoy.com. It is a great resource. Additionally, Joy is now offering even more, which is described below:

> To bring a true "dose of JOY" to those fighting cancer and those supporting them, Joy is also providing something very unique. Her book already lists more than twenty-five pages of helpful resources. Now you can sign-up to receive this information in short video messages at www.cancerwithjoy.com Joy *shows* you around the resources that she shares in her book, saving you tremendous amounts of time and energy trying to find your way around these helpful resources. Instead of just telling you to visit www.cancer.net (as an example), each short video shows you around a different resource's website. The best part is you can watch them from your hospital bed, and be helped and inspired even if you can't travel to see Joy speak live. I encourage you to check out this unique offering of videos from Joy!

Survival Tips

- Take a break; you don't have to learn it all today.
- Take a walk; notice the birds.
- Resist. Resist the urge to proceed headlong into anything until you have considered the facts and options. While it is important that treatment begins soon, remember the situation didn't get

there overnight, and a day or two to gather your wits and the facts won't matter.

- Read. Read pamphlets, books, and trusted websites. Search for blogs that address the issue. Often your doctor will be able to provide you with written material that describes the cancer that you have, the treatment options, and what to expect. Some may have a DVD that you can take home and watch. As you gain information, you may identify new questions. These will be items to write down and ask your doctor at the next visit. When you begin to learn, you will also find out you are not alone.
- Respect your loved one's right not to want to know right now.
- Talk to a trusted friend. Tell them you need to just talk about what you are learning. They will be glad to know they don't have to have answers.

What a Friend Can Do to Help

- Listen, listen, listen. Your friend or family member is going through a time of learning a lot of new information. Sometimes we learn best by teaching others. You can help a great deal if you will simply be willing to listen as they explain to you what is happening. Ask good questions—ones that clarify information such as, "Can you explain again how the treatment process will work?" Also ask questions that will help process and clarify decisions and emotions, such as, "How are you feeling about the treatment that has been suggested?"
- Save your advice and war stories for another time. If asked, share your experience briefly, focusing on the positives. Your friend simply does not have the interest, stamina, or need right now to focus on all the things that may have gone wrong in your situation. Certainly, if you learned something that will be helpful, share it, but do so briefly and positively. Do remember that though similar, every situation is different, and it is their doctor, not you, that knows the specifics of what is happening to them.

Kubler-Ross Stages of Grief

Denial: "This cannot happen to me!"

Anger: "Why did this happen to me? Who's to blame for this?"

Bargaining: "If you'll just let me live until my daughter's wedding, I'll do anything."

Depression: "I am too sad to do anything."

Acceptance: "I'm at peace with what is coming."

- Learn about the grieving process. Even now, everyone involved in this illness is beginning to face loss. It may be as simple as the loss of time to office visits or tests. It may be as huge as a diagnosis of terminal illness. Grief begins now. Sometimes grief is messy. You may be called upon to be patient, supportive, and forgiving. Knowing about the process can be helpful.

FEEL—FELT—FOUND

I can understand how you feel…

I felt _____ when _____.

But I found _____.

- Feel—felt—found. Use this guide to respond in a way that is helpful.
  1. Name the feeling that you see or hear and then voice understanding and acceptance of the feeling. *I can understand how you feel _____.*
  2. Relate very briefly a time when you also felt that feeling. *I felt that way too when _____.*
  3. Suggest an alternative that might be helpful. *But I found that _____.*

An example: "*I can understand that you feel angry; I felt that way when I lost my mother. I found that talking about it helped.*"

- Offer concrete help. Think about the problems that would exist for you if you were in that situation, decide what you would be willing to do to help, and offer it. "I could keep your dog for few days" is so much better than "let me know if I can do anything."
- Offer a diversion: a cup of coffee, a trip to the local drive-in for a shake.
- Forgive and be patient when your friend has a one track mind.
- Pray. Prayer moves the hand of God, and right now, your friend or family member could use some movement, so be part of the solution.

Points to Ponder

I am the Lord your God, who teaches you what is best for you, who directs you in the way you should go.
—**Isaiah 48:17**

It's when we become deaf to God's Word that it presents a problem to us. When we fail to stay close to His Word and focused on him, His messages to us go unnoticed.

But where do I read? What if His answer is in Matthew and I am reading in John? I have struggled with this question at times. The answer is really pretty simple, just read.

Unlike any other book that you will ever read or own, the Bible is a living book, it can speak to you wherever you happen to be. It will be less difficult, however, if you just develop a daily habit and follow some kind of a plan.

One way to do this is to find a devotional book or Bible study that you just work through every day.

A second way is to use the following: Read at least one of the Psalms every day. Start at the beginning, read through, and when you get to the end start over.

Each day, read the chapter of Proverbs that corresponds to the date. Proverbs has thirty-one chapters. In a month's time you will have read the entire book. One thing I like to do is to put a date or check mark by the verse in the chapter that stood out the most. Sometimes there will be only one, sometimes several. When I come to that chapter month after month, I am always surprised that the verse that meant so much last month says nothing this month, but another one seems to be shouting. That's God. Stop and consider that verse. Maybe even write it on a small card and carry it with you. Meditate on it throughout the day and let God put its meaning for you in your heart.

If you are a new Christian, or new to Bible reading, consider adding the book of John in the New Testament to what you are reading. It is the fourth book in the New Testament and one of the gospels that tells the story of Jesus's life on this earth, his teachings, and miracles.

Part Two

Negotiating the Medical World

Waiting

This magazine, I've seen before.
Is that the same family over there that I saw yesterday?
Alcohol from the lab nearby tickles my nose.
It mixes with the smell of fresh brewed coffee,
made by the hospital volunteer.
I am silent, waiting.
Yet all around me busy people don't seem to notice.
Inside, my mind goes places I don't want to be.
Endless hours it seems.
Today it is a PET scan,
Yesterday, the lab.
Why all these tests.
I just want answers.
Instead,
I wait.

Chapter Three

Recruiting the Medical Team

· ·

Ruth was her name. She was the surgeon's nurse. In the three years I received care in their office, she never again answered the phone. But that day she did, answered, listened, and acted. I saw the doctor three days later.

· ·

Two weeks, thirteen days to be exact, after my husband lost his battle with cancer, I found a lump in my breast; a lump which ultimately turned out to be cancerous. My first reaction was to go to the medical office, the nurse practitioner who, along with our oncologist, had become my medical rock and friend throughout the years of my husband's treatment.

I had seen her eleven days earlier at the funeral home. Now I sat holding my breath as she examined my find.

Later, when the diagnosis was confirmed, my sons, having just lost their father, insisted this time we get advice from a major cancer center before proceeding.

Living in the Midwest, our first thought and choice was MD Anderson in Texas, so that's where I began. Roadblocks immediately were evident. After several calls, it seemed I would have to wait six weeks to even see a doctor there.

The nurse practitioner suggested a doctor at Kansas University Medical Center, a surgeon who specialized in breast cancer. I made the call. What happened next can only be explained as the hand of God directing my care.

The call was answered on the first attempt by the surgeon's nurse. It was not her job to answer the phone and on other occasions when I called, she never answered it. Over the next years I found her to be extremely busy and difficult to connect with, but that day she was the one I talked to. Ruth listened, asked questions, and acted. I saw the surgeon three days later. I have since come to realize she was used of God that day to open the treatment door He had chosen for me.

Pray First for Wisdom and Guidance

In all the seeking and looking for the right medical team, I can now look back and see how God's guiding hand directed us to the right people, to the right place, exactly on time. Never is there a time to practice 1 Thessalonians 5:17's *pray without ceasing* more than now.

God knows exactly who is best involved with your situation. Perhaps it is a physician who just learned of a new way to treat your type of cancer. It may be the physician is not the issue, but it is the receptionist at a particular clinic that He knows will take a special interest in scheduling your appointment at just the right time. Maybe it's the building janitor standing by the elevator that will encourage you just when you need it most. God knows. Your first job is to get yourself situated so you are hearing and heeding His direction.

Note: If you are reading this and there has never been a time when you asked the Lord Jesus to come into your life and take over, that is the first step. Before you go further, read *What the Bible Says* in the *Afterword*. Listening is not an easy job, and it's impossible if you don't have access to the music.

Where Do I Start?

If you have been seeing a primary physician for your ongoing health care needs, this is the place to start. This is the doctor who knows you best. Before concerns present themselves, make regular checkups a part of your health care regimen. Visit your doctor for yearly checks. Go when you are well. Many screening tests might be skewed if you are ill and/or on medications. At this appointment, remind the doctor of any diseases prevalent in your family history.

I suspect you might be thinking, *I told them that when I first started seeing them.* While it is true this information is probably in your record, it's likely pages down, and you are not his/her only patient. Our parents lived in an age when the doctor they saw was the one who also cared for Mom and Dad, Grandma and Grandpa, and all their siblings. Of course he knew the family history. He lived it with them; that isn't the case today. So, don't expect your doctor to be God. There is only one of those and he/she isn't it.

Begin now to take charge of your health. At your yearly appointment, don't be shy. Tell him/her of any symptoms and concerns. Remind him of your family history. Ask whether there are recommended screenings that you, at your age, given your family history, should have.

Referral to a Specialist

Indicators of concerns will likely result in your being referred to a specialist. You have a right and responsibility to be involved in the choice. Listen to your doctor. Ask questions: What is their experience? Will my insurance plan cover his/her services or will I have to pay extra? What other choices are available? Do you suspect cancer, and if so, should I see an oncologist first? (See *Questions to Ask Your Doctor* in the Appendix).

When you see the specialist, understand they will not immediately have an answer to that most pressing question in your mind. "Do I have cancer and am I going to die?" They should be able and willing to talk with you about possibilities, evaluation tests, and options for evaluations. I do not think it is premature, even at this first appointment to ask about who and where he would likely recommend if your situation warrants referral to a national cancer center. You will not offend them. A good doctor will be the first to suggest a referral or second opinions if he believes it will be helpful. In my case, I consulted an oncologist at a major cancer center, and he worked with my oncologist at home so that I received the best of both.

National Cancer Centers

A National Cancer Center is a hospital or research facility that has met rigorous guidelines in the areas of diagnosis, treatment, and research. It is here the latest treatments are being developed. It is here you would go to be included in a research trial. I don't know that it is always necessary to seek such a center for treatment. If your doctors have determined that your cancer is a common type, in an early stage, you will likely not benefit greatly by going to a major center. If, however, your cancer is an unusual type, advancing, or has other complicating factors, this might be a good choice. It is alright, and even best, to talk with your current doctor about this possibility. They will give you their opinion. They will work with those teams if you go.

It's Not Just About the Doctor— Finding the Right Medical Team

When you are dealing with an ongoing, serious illness, you will see a multitude of people. During the months of my cancer treatment, many physicians were involved in my care. Many I never saw. They were the pathologists, radiologists, anesthesiologists, etc., who looked at my X-rays, PET scans, CT scans, bone scans, MRIs, MUGA Scans, blood and tissue samples, and so on.

Although there were some I never met, some of the doctors, nurses, and staff became almost like family. They saw us at our worst, cared for us when we couldn't care for ourselves, calmed our fears, and cheered us on. They were not, however, in every case, the first doctor we saw. Sometimes change is needed, and if it doesn't seem like the team you have "fits," don't be afraid to do so. This is a long journey and it's kind of like marriage—it is a whole lot more fun if you like each other.

We were well into our second year of my husband's treatment before we knew he had rectal cancer, not colon cancer, and one meaning of this was that metastasis (spreading to other locations) was more likely to be to the lungs not the liver. The surgeon had told me, initially, not to worry if the cancer spread to the liver because there were treatments. Three months after the original diagnosis, a PET scan showed "hot spots" in the lungs. I was confused.

Our questions were answered with short tentative replies and little information. God apparently knew change was needed. On one occasion, we were scheduled to get test results but our regular doctor was out of town. At this visit, we saw the doctor who was to become our rock.

The forty-five minute appointment changed our direction. Our whys were answered with detailed information. This doctor apparently believed "a picture was worth a thousand words." We spent the appointment huddled around the exam table instead of on it. An elaborate, hand drawn diagram, yes, using the exam table paper, allowed us to fully understand what and why things had gone as they had. On our trip home, we discussed changing doctors. Some people don't need to know all the specifics, and my husband was a bit that way. I, on the other hand, in addition to being an RN, am a "thinker."

Thinkers need to know, understand, talk through, and ask a lot of questions. Changing oncologists in mid-stream wasn't in our plan, but it did end up being right. The new doctor treated my husband carefully and thoroughly, all the while, providing me, the nurse/wife with the information I needed and wanted.

Three years later, in another forty-five minute appointment, this same doctor addressed my physical, mental, and emotional issues. It was eighteen months past my husband's death. I had completed my own year-long cancer treatment and had gone in for a routine follow-up appointment. I was struggling, not with the cancer, but with how to survive. I was cancer free, but still physically weak. I was eighteen months into widowhood but, because of my own disease, was just beginning to truly grieve. I was sure something was wrong—I thought I should be better by now and I was pushing frantically to be okay. Fatigue discouraged me.

His prescription that day was far better than any medication I could have received. "Do what you have to do in the morning, eat lunch, take a one hour rest/nap, and in the afternoon, do only what you want to do." It was a miracle cure for my frantic attempt to find normal. I still use that plan today.

Who is on Your Team?

Primary Physician
We found, in the active stages of treatment, our primary physician kind of just stood on the sideline. But like a good coach, he offered direction and encouragement when needed.

Oncologist
This is the specialist who will guide your cancer treatment team. It is important he/she knows about your particular type of cancer, keeps up-to-date on changing treatment recommendations, welcomes your request for a second opinion, or suggests it, and lastly communicates well. Both you and your doctor will have lots of questions to answer and decisions to make. There are many decisions in cancer treatment and some of them will be yours alone. Choose a doctor who will listen, hear, teach, and guide.

Radiologist

These specialists will read your X-rays and scans, and if needed, plan and supervise radiation treatments. There will likely be several, many you may never see. They are kind of like those programs that run your computer. You don't really ever see or think about them, but they are essential if things are to be done correctly.

Cardiologist

Even if you have no previous heart problems, it is not unlikely that you will end up with one of these on your team. Some cancer drugs can be very hard on the heart and require special monitoring to assure that you are treated with the fewest possible side effects. They may monitor you even after the chemotherapy treatments are completed to assure any possible problems are recognized and treated. In treating his colon cancer, my husband did not incur any cardiac side effects. One of the drugs that I took for breast cancer, however, was known to have cardiac side effects. During the fourth treatment round, I had an episode of tachycardia (rapid heart rate) that resulted in hospitalization—and the acquisition of yet another physician, a cardiologist, on my treatment team.

Pathologist

This specialist is in the lab and is vital to the diagnosis. They look at the tissue samples and determine the type and extent of the disease.

Nurse Practitioner

These are RNs who have advanced training and licensure to provide medical interventions. They work directly with the physician in providing your care and are a priceless addition to your team; one of their specialties is anticipating, treating, and managing side effects.

Chemotherapy Nurses

These are the people who will be in the trenches with you, so to speak. They are skilled at administering the drugs and monitoring the side effects. They are like moms who seem to have eyes in the back of their heads when it comes to recognizing problems, alerting the doctor, and intervening on your behalf. They seem to have God's healing touch. I don't know, maybe they really are angels in disguise.

Survival Tips

- Begin a journal of your experiences and appointments. Record the tests you have, your symptoms, feelings, and questions.
- Ask others who have experienced similar situations for recommendations.
- Don't be afraid to see your first appointment as an interview. Ask questions.

What a Friend Can Do to Help

- Continue to pray. Don't let up. Satan would like to discourage all of you. It's a fight and your help is needed.
- Develop a system of praying for others. I have discovered that it can be very overwhelming to remember who I need to be lifting before the Father's throne. I have adopted the habit of pausing to pray for someone who I know is ill or has a special need, whenever I see their name, whether on Facebook, in a blog, or on a prayer list. I find I pray more regularly for others with this method.

Points to Ponder

Yea, though I walk through the valley of the shadow of death, I will fear no evil: for thou art with me; thy rod and thy staff they comfort me. Thou preparest a table

before me in the presence of mine enemies: thou anointest
my head with oil; my cup runneth over.

—Psalm 23:4–5

In biblical times it was the custom to invite a passing stranger to sit and dine with you. A little known custom was this: when it came time to end the meal, a cup, full and running over, was signal to the guest that they were welcome to stay the night. God tells us in this psalm that He has filled our cup to overflowing and we can stay. So sit with Him. Walk with Him. Stay. Let Him be your friend through the coming days.

Chapter Four

Tests, Procedures, and Definitions

∙∙∙∙∙∙∙∙∙∙∙∙∙∙∙∙∙∙∙∙∙∙∙∙∙∙∙∙∙∙∙∙

I wanted answers,
but all they had were questions.

∙∙∙∙∙∙∙∙∙∙∙∙∙∙∙∙∙∙∙∙∙∙∙∙∙∙∙∙∙∙∙∙

What Happens Next?

By this time in your journey, if you have already received a diagnosis, you have been poked and prodded until it seems like a normal part of your day. What used to be a dreaded procedure has become nearly boring. That may be an exaggeration, but you get the point.

Even as a nurse, I was overwhelmed by the names and types of tests. I was well down the road before I had a good understanding of why this or that test was ordered. So, it's okay if you need to take a deep breath and not read this whole chapter in one sitting. In fact, you may not want to read it at all, at least right now. Use it as a reference when you need it. When you are ready, or need it, specific information will be in two places.

In this chapter, I will begin at the beginning and walk through the process, focusing on those tests more commonly used and why. Many of the tests may be repeated throughout the treatment experience. Initially, the testing is done for the purpose of diagnosing the problem. Later, tests are used to monitor the effectiveness of treatment and watch for the return of the disease once treatment is finished. Currently, five years past my own treatment for breast cancer, I still see my doctor every six months for exam and lab work. One of those labs monitors the marker for breast cancer.

Before: A Routine Physical

When you see your physician for a routine physical, he will ask you questions. It will be good if you prepare for the visit by making a list of the things you want to ask also.

The doctor will end the visit with a physical examination. He, or his nurse, will take your blood pressure, pulse, and temperature. The doctor may ask you to change into an exam gown. This will allow him to palpate or feel for any lumps, bumps, or masses. Typically, a routine exam will include a look into your eyes, ears, nose, and throat. He will ask you to swallow while he palpates your neck area. He will be watching for swelling that could indicate your thyroid is not functioning correctly or that your lymph glands are enlarged. He will also be looking for other signs of swelling, especially in your feet or legs, which could indicate a problem with your circulation. He will examine your belly for anything that appears abnormal. If you are a female, a breast exam and a pelvic exam are in order. If a male, the doctor will check for prostate or hernia problems. While not pleasant, these exams may save your life.

It is quite normal for the doctor to order other tests to be sure things are going well on the inside. These are screening tests. Abnormalities can signal the need to check further. They also provide a baseline for later follow-ups.

Labs

There are literally hundreds of tests that can be done on blood, tissue, and other body fluids. Here are some of the more common tests:

- CBC: The doctor will check your red and white cell count. Doing this allows him to check many things. Commonly, he is looking to see if you are anemic (low hemoglobin), or have signs of infection (a high white blood cell count).
- Chemistry Panel: Chemistry panels are groups of tests that examine the electrolytes in your body. Electrolytes are the minerals, such as potassium, sodium, calcium, magnesium, and other substances that keep things running right. Chemistry panels can also check liver and kidney functioning.
- Urinalysis: The doctor may want to examine a urine specimen. From it he can detect signs of infections, problems with your sugar metabolism, and your kidney functioning. He can also tell if you are dehydrated.

Electrocardiogram (EKG or ECG):

Your doctor may order an EKG. This test records the electrical activity of the heart and is used in diagnosing some heart abnormalities.

Colonoscopy

I saved this one until last. If your doctor doesn't suggest it and you are age fifty or older, or if you are younger with a family history of colon cancer, you must suggest it. Everyone dreads this test. In reality, the prep is mildly bothersome, the IV to provide sedation is a little pin prick, and the next thing you know, the test is over. Actually, it might be the first good nap you've had in a long time!

According to the American Cancer Society, a colonoscopy, while it will take about twenty-four hours of your time between prep and procedure, can often find colorectal cancer early when there is about a 75% chance of cure. Often, it is prevented entirely because precancerous polyps are found and removed. The other end of that spectrum, stage four colorectal cancer has about a 6% survival rate. In between that are various stages of disease and treatment, most of which is no fun at all. So twenty-four hours … your life … twenty-four hours … your life … hmmm, hard choice isn't it?

Symptoms Signal an Alarm— See your Regular Doctor First

Okay, so the day comes when you decide it's time to see a doctor because of concerning symptoms. Go prepared. Make a list of the symptoms you are experiencing and the questions you want to ask. Do not leave out anything just because it doesn't seem worth mentioning. It may be a minor thing, but coupled with other symptoms it may give clues to what is wrong. If you will remember in my earlier account of our situation, not until I had that last piece of the puzzle, did it trigger the understanding of what might be wrong.

Your doctor may order some tests. Whether or not he does so will depend partially on how long it has been since you had regular testing. The symptoms you have may lead him to order others.

It may be your doctor will immediately refer you to a specialist. That could be because he suspects a problem, but it may also be simply because your symptoms are out of his area of expertise. So don't fear (remember that if you do it's God's heads up) and follow through.

We actually experienced both. My husband was immediately referred to a surgeon, I on the other hand was sent for a mammogram. Incidentally, I was one month overdue for one. A close friend delayed a bit longer. Though she fought valiantly, the delay ultimately cost her life.

Referred: Seeing the Specialist

In both cases, we were first referred to a surgeon. That is a usual course of action. Maybe that is alright, but as I look back, I wish we had first consulted an oncologist. I understand that nobody wants to say, or hear, the word cancer. Still, before any surgery is done, be sure. It is not whether or not surgery is needed; it's a matter of the timing. Sometimes, it is better to have treatment before the surgery takes place. Whoever you see first, remember knowledge is power. Ask questions, such as: What do you suspect is wrong? If it turns out I have cancer, would it be advisable to consult with an oncologist before I have the surgery? What are my treatment options? What are the advantages and disadvantages of either route? Are there tests that should be done first to help establish a treatment plan?

Diagnostic Tests and Exams

The following are tests that are routinely done in the diagnosis and treatment stages of cancer.

X-Ray. These are usually painless and require that you sit, stand, or lay on a table and an X-ray beam is momentarily sent from the machine to the plate containing film. This is somewhat like an old fashioned photo and negative. A radiologist will read the X-ray to see if the picture on the film looks like he would expect in a normal situation free of disease or fractures. He looks for shadows, light or dark areas that should be just the opposite. X-rays are a beginning, but usually do not provide the depth of information gained from other scans. It is a screening tool. The advantage of X-ray is that it is quick, available, and relatively inexpensive. Additionally, an X-ray done for another purpose such as checking for bone fractures or pneumonia, may provide the first clue that a cancer might be present.

Sonograms. Sonograms are minimally invasive tests that are done by passing a specialized instrument over an area of the body after an odorless, colorless gel is applied to the area. Sound waves are emitted and bounce back to provide an X-ray like picture. A sonogram is not painful and usually is readily available.

Body Scans. In the diagnosis and monitoring of disease, there are several scans that are routinely used. Easily searched on the Internet, these scans can still remain confusing. The description here, while not technical and complete, will give you a simple description of what happens and what the scans are used for.

Bone Scan. Two types of bone scans may be done.

- Bone Density Scan (DXA). This is a quick and painless scan that measures bone mineral density. It is used to diagnose and monitor osteoporosis. I had the scan done to provide a baseline prior to beginning chemo drugs that could cause bone loss. It continues to be part of my follow-up care.

- Nuclear Medicine Scan. This scan will use an injection of a nuclear isotope to diagnose and track several types of bone disease. It may be done if you have unexplained skeletal pain suggesting bone loss, bone infection, or a bone injury undetectable on a standard X-ray.

This scan is also used to detect cancer that has spread (metastasized) to the bone from a tumor that started in a different organ, such as the breast or prostate. It may also detect some abnormalities related to leukemia and lymphoma.

CT Scans—Computed Tomography (also called CAT Scan). This scan is done by lying flat and without moving being transported into the CT scanner. It takes many X-ray pictures which are then converted to computer images. It visualizes both soft tissue and bone and can be assembled into 3-D images. CT scans are like an X-ray in that an abnormality is seen as an area that is white when it should be black or vice-versa. The difference is that the CT scanner takes many pictures. These pictures show cross sections of the body in many thin layers, much as if you sliced a carrot into very thin carrot coins. CTs may be done with or without contrast.

In either case, you will be placed on a flat surface and will need to lie still for several minutes. The scan itself is painless, but having to lie still may be uncomfortable if you are anxious or have chronic pain. If you are concerned about this, talk to your doctor about the possibility of taking medication before the procedure to help calm your nerves or lessen the discomfort.

The flat surface that you are laying on will move slowly into the scanner tunnel, which is about twenty-four inches across. Unless you are having a CT of your head, it will remain outside the scanner. You will hear clicking and whirring noises. After having several scans, I found that it helped if I just closed my eyes and used the time to pray for all the people who were caring for me; the doctors, nurses, technicians, my family, and friends. The scan was almost always over before I could get through my list. I kind of knew, however, that God would finish the list, even when I was interrupted by the technician announcing, "All through."

PET—Positron Emission Tomography. Once in the scanner, the PET scan and CT scan are nearly identical in how you will be positioned, what you will hear, and feel. The difference is that the PET scan is a nuclear medicine procedure. You will be given a small amount of radioactive material in a highly concentrated sugar solution. Because the body uses sugar for energy, the solution will migrate to areas of the body where there is a lot of metabolic activity. Cancer cells are growing at a faster rate than normal cells. Because of this they will draw the radioactive sugar substance to the site and the scanner will then see them. These show up on the scans as "hot spots" and look a bit like what happens when the flash of a camera catches a shiny object and makes a white spot on the photo. You will be asked to restrict your intake of sugary foods and drinks for a period of time before the scan. It is very important that you comply with this request. Doing so will reduce the amount of sugar metabolism going on in your body at the time of the scan, making the radioactive sugar substance more prominent. When reading the scan, the doctor will look for such activity in areas where it shouldn't be.

PET Scans are done in similar slices as the CT, except they run lengthwise instead of crosswise, as if you were cutting the carrot lengthwise into long thin slices, instead of crosswise into coins. Because it is looking at cellular activity, a PET scan may detect the early onset of disease before it is evident on other imaging tests such as CT or MRI.

I always took a book or magazine to read when I was having a PET scan. After you have been given the radioactive material, you will need to wait about 45 minutes to an hour to allow it to circulate in your body, usually in a comfy recliner, with an optional blanket to keep you warm. I actually kind of looked forward to that little period of imposed relaxation, where no phones or people interrupted.

In the scanner, I again used the time to pray for my caregivers. All in all, it wasn't the worst way to spend a morning.

MRI—Magnetic Resonance Imaging. This test using magnetic energy radio frequency pulses. It's not painful at all, but it is noisy. Often earplugs are used. Otherwise, it is very similar to the CT scan. It does take a bit longer. In some cases, particularly with soft tissue structures of the body, an MRI is more helpful in accurately diagnosing and evaluating the characteristics of a tumor or lesion.

A Note about the Future

Even as I write, things are changing as new, different, and more sophisticated evaluation and treatment options become available. New combinations of CT, PET, and MRI are on the horizon and being used in combination to provide better, quicker, noninvasive diagnosis. I recommend visiting www.Radiologyinfo.org for further descriptions and insights.

Seeing the Oncologist

The Oncologist may repeat many of the tests and exams done earlier. It is always best to have two opinions and this is an area where twice is good. One of the things I believe we all need to remember is no doctor can know everything. Having a second doctor find something suspicious is not a sign of malpractice. It is a sign that your doctors are human—or that in the time elapsed between the two visits, a lump, bump, or swelling has grown to where it is large enough to feel.

It is helpful in moving things along for the specialist to have access to any tests that have already been done. The lab or your physician can send the records or you can hand carry them yourself. I prefer the later. In the medical records chapter, I will talk more about record keeping. For now, just let me say, when you hand carry your records to the specialist there will never be a delay because the records haven't yet arrived.

On one particular occasion, I traveled one hundred fifty miles and was being admitted for surgery, only to hear from the nurse that my preoperative lab work had not arrived from my home laboratory. I was able to produce them, because I had gone to the lab, gotten the results, and filed them in my binder. The surgery, which might have been delayed or postponed, proceeded as scheduled.

The oncologist will look at all the test results and scans that you or your regular doctor has provided to him. He may order more tests. There seem to be a few that are pretty standard in the diagnostic realm. Earlier, I discussed the differences in people and how and why we want different amounts of information. Whatever it is for you and your loved one, seek out your medical team for answers. I have high praises for the team that coupled with us in our cancer fight. You deserve that too. Seek it. Ask the doctor to explain what he is ordering a test and why. It is good to begin gaining the knowledge about what is happening from the very beginning. When tests are done, obtain a copy, and file it in your medical record binder.

Tumor Markers

This is a lab test done on blood, urine, stool, or other bodily fluids. Most are done on blood samples. Without meaning to scare you, get used to the needle sticks. They are just part of the territory. One day you will look back and say, "I can't believe I was so upset over a little needle stick."

Tumor marker results are used in several ways:

- To help diagnose cancer
- To help predict a patient's response to certain cancer therapies
- To check a patient's response to treatment
- To determine cancer reoccurrence

More than twenty tumor markers are currently in use. Some may even be done as part of a routine physical. The PSA test is an example.

For years, it has been widely used to screen for prostate cancer. Most routine lab work done on men over the age of fifty includes this valuable screening test.

Other tumor markers are monitored only after a diagnosis is made and are used for monitoring treatment effectiveness. CEA is one such marker. It is used to monitor treatment effectiveness and reoccurrence with colorectal or breast cancer. There is not a universal tumor marker. There are also limitations as to their usefulness since some noncancerous conditions can cause these levels to increase. Additionally, two people with the same type of cancer may have very different levels of the specific marker associated with that particular type of cancer. Often the usefulness is not in the level itself but in the changes in the level as treatment progresses. And there are some cancer types for which no markers have been identified.

Staging

Staging is a term used to describe the determination of how far the cancer has progressed. Generally it includes a rating from 0 to IV (expressed in Roman Numerals) and may have A-C levels within the numbered stage. Other factors may be included. Because staging criteria may be applied differently with each type of cancer, it is necessary to research the staging as it applies to your particular type of cancer.

Survival Tips

- Consider having someone go with you to appointments where you know you will be getting test results or will be making decisions about what to do next. All that information can be overwhelming and it helps to have someone who will just sit back with a pen and paper and take notes.
- Keep a notebook that has all your questions and answers. Write the questions down as they occur to you. Don't wait until you are sitting in the waiting room to think of all you want or need to know. If you have someone with you who will just take notes,

give them your notebook. Let them record the answers right there. They can also watch and prompt you if you forget to ask a question that you have written down.

- When possible, schedule appointments when it is most convenient for you. I had one surgeon who was two hours away. Appointments at eight in the morning would have been a nightmare. If, however, I scheduled the appointment for right after lunch, I had time to have a leisurely drive there, grab a bite of lunch and, if I felt up to it, I still had time to indulge my shopping habit before returning home.

- Carry a book or magazine with you. Turn waiting into a mini retreat. It's easy to feel guilty about time to yourself when you have the responsibilities that go with caregiving. Snuggling in with a good book, even if it is in the waiting room chair, can feel like a guilt-free indulgence if you let it. Many waiting rooms have coffee and even snacks, especially if they are oncology centers.

What a Friend Can Do to Help

- Offer to go along or drive to the appointment. Offer to even attend and take notes (see the first point above).
- If asked, don't lie about a test you know to be unpleasant, but don't exaggerate it either.
- If not asked, don't offer information or advice. Be considerate of the person's right to have information at their pace, not yours. We all accept reality differently and in different time frames. When they are ready to know, they will ask.

Points to Ponder

> *Be strong and of a good courage, fear not, nor be afraid of them: for the lord thy god, he it is that doth go with thee; he will not fail thee, nor forsake thee.*
>
> **—Deuteronomy 31:6**

How bad is it—really?

Have you ever known anybody who was the queen of *Ain't it Awful?* I have. A conversation with them goes something like this:

You: "Well, good morning, how are you?"

Ain't it Awful: "Oh, just horrible. I got up too late and spilled my coffee on my shirt and had to change it and then I got behind someone going so slow I was even later, and then the rain started and I got wet."

Quite frequently, Ain't it Awful is the first one to tell you about the test you are scheduled to have. It's not pretty.

You: "Yes, I am having a PET scan next week."

Ain't it Awful: "Oh my, I remember when I had that test. It was awful. I had to eat all this crazy food before and then they couldn't get the IV started and it was awful. They kept sticking me and sticking me, and then I had to sit in this awful little room, and all the time I was dreading the test."

It's likely not every test, procedure, and treatment is going to be totally pleasant. Sometimes things are awkward, uncomfortable, a little painful, or otherwise difficult. You will survive. Much of the time it is attitude that makes the difference. Being anxious, fearful, and angry will make it more difficult. In Deuteronomy 31:6 we are instructed to act differently. God has never told us we would never have pain or discomfort. He has, however, promised He will be with us when we do. Trust Him and do not fear. Focus your attention on Him and not the procedure.

Chapter Five

Medical Records
and Insurance

· ·

One day several months following my year
of treatment for breast cancer, I found myself
sorting through the insurance records and billing
statements. Noting a physician's name that was
unfamiliar, I began to look, and count. Twenty-
six different physicians had billed my insurance
during that year. Most I never saw or knew.
Nevertheless they had somehow played a part in
my treatment or care.

· ·

Records

Your Medical Records/Your Rights

The Privacy Rule gives you, with few exceptions, the right to inspect, review, and receive a copy of your medical records and billing records that are held by health plans and health care providers covered by the Privacy Rule. However, only you or your <u>personal representative</u> has the right to access your records. You will need to sign a release of information prior to them receiving a copy. A full explanation of the Privacy Rule may be found on the Health and Human Services website at <u>www.hhs.gov</u>.

Keep a copy of your medical records. Start a file now. Get a copy of every medical record from all sources. In four years of cancer treatment, there were several times that treatment or consultation would have been delayed had we not had a copy of the needed record.

Be kind to the people who manage the paper, they are just doing their job. It is very tempting to become short tempered with medical personnel who insist on following the letter of the law when it comes to releasing information. Resist. They are doing the right thing. They are following their agency's guidelines. They are complying with federal law. More importantly, their diligence assures you that the mound of records that your illness is generating remains private. Thank them!

How to Organize a Medical Record Binder

There are several ways you can keep your records organized. Which one you choose will depend on your personal style and desire.

1. Chronological Order
    a. Method: Using a three-hole punch, put holes in the record and insert in a three-ring notebook. Put it in date order with the newest on the top.
    b. Advantage(s)
        i. Easiest to maintain
        ii. Current record always on top

      c. Disadvantage(s)

         i. Diagnostic reports harder to find

2. Sections

      a. Method: Add divider sections to a three-ring notebook and file records behind the appropriate divider with the most current on top. Suggested divisions are:

         i. History & physicals, treatment summaries, consult reports

         ii. Diagnostic testing (excluding laboratories)

         iii. Laboratory results (if desired, you could subdivide these by type)

         iv. Other records

      b. Advantage(s)

         i. Specific reports are easier to find

      c. Disadvantage(s)

         i. More time consuming to maintain

3. Expandable file folder

      a. Method: Using an expandable file folder, label each section, and file records in the appropriate place.

      b. Advantage(s)

         i. Easier to transport

         ii. Easy to maintain

      c. Disadvantage(s)

         i. Records can become mixed up or misplaced more easily

         ii. Must be removed to be read

4. Electronic Records

      a. Method: The newest method of record keeping is to receive your records electronically. If you do this, your records will be placed on a disc so that you may load them on your own computer, or hand-carry to another person. A provider may also be able to e-mail your records to you. Between physicians, most records are now transmitted electronically. Consents to do so are normally signed by you on your initial visit to the provider.

    b. Advantage(s)

        i.   Decreased paper to maintain and store

        ii. Easy to organize if you are computer savvy

    c. Disadvantage(s)

        i.   Must have a computer to view them

Dealing with Insurance and Medical Bills

I had quit a job where I had good insurance to pursue a home business opportunity. It was not a concern because my husband's insurance through his job was good. Still, in January of 2004, my husband began saying to me, "I think you should go back to work where you have insurance." He didn't harp on it, but about once a month or so he would mention it. Five months passed and while visiting with a friend who was also a nurse, a job opportunity presented itself and I took it. I started full time in June of 2004. In October of that same year, my husband was diagnosed with cancer and never worked again. We would have been without insurance, had God not orchestrated my return to employment.

Still, one of the most ongoing frustrations with chronic illness is the paperwork that arrives in your mail box almost daily. It is good to begin a system of dealing with it from the beginning. In most cases you won't need to do anything with most of it, however, occasionally you will so it's best to keep it all at least for a while.

What follows is a paper sorting method I use that works for me. It includes all paper that I deal with, not just mail.

On arrival, all mail goes in one place. Get a basket or a box or a drawer, and just put it there. Add to it the receipts from your purse, pictures the grandkids draw, and other papers that migrate to your home.

When you are ready to deal with it, you need a trash can, two storage boxes, and a filing tray marked IN.

Take things out of the basket one at a time and deal with it completely. Throw junk mail, outside envelopes, and anything else you don't need in the trash. For me, a successful paper sort is a full trash can, it's almost as good as chocolate.

If you need to keep a paper, it goes one of three places.

- Box one: I might need this, I don't think so, but I better keep it a while just in case. An example here might be the scheduling papers you got for the CT scan next week, you've already put it on your calendar and know what to do, but just in case.
- Box two: This is a tax receipt that I need to keep. The bill from the motel you stayed in when you went to the cancer center would be an example.
- File Tray: This is a record that I need to keep indefinitely. Examples might be the picture your granddaughter drew that was especially meaningful, the discharge summary from a recent hospital stay, improvements made to property you own, etc.

Trash is emptied when you are finished with each sort.

Box One, when full, is closed, dated to discard in six months (put the actual discard date on it, i.e., "Discard on June 1, 20XX"), and stored in an out of the way but accessible place that you routinely check for discards, maybe a garage shelf.

Box Two contains all of the records you need to keep for tax purposes. I add an extra step in here so that I do not have to deal with all of the paper at the end of the year. I have a scanner filing program. Before papers go in the box, I scan them and then I have a digital image and I don't have to deal with paper later. It's a new program, but as I trust it more, most of the paper I keep can be thrown away. For now, I just keep it all. If you do not use such a program, you could do the same thing with even a simple three ring notebook. Just write down the figures you need at the end of the year, put the paper in the box and store it. The box should be big enough to hold all of a calendar year's papers. When you are done with them, seal, and label "Discard in seven years (date)." They also go in that storage spot.

Keep what is left. File them in your file drawer by category.

Insurance

Private Insurance and Medicare

For the most part, we had few insurance problems. There were a few glitches that I suspect could be common ones. I will describe them here.

1. Non-covered medications and treatments. There were only a couple of times that this occurred for us. In both cases, the physician or nurse practitioner communicated directly with the insurance company to provide the information needed to qualify them as necessary. This would always be the first avenue. Talk to your physician. In some cases, an alternate medication may work just as well and be covered without question. In others, the physician can provide information that explains why you need to have the non-covered medication and it may be approved for payment.

2. Treatments, tests, or visits that were not covered by the insurance company and were not paid. This only happened once in our experience. A provider billed separately for a visit and a test when the contract with the insurance company stated that only one charge would be paid. I don't think this was an attempt to fraud. I think it was an honest billing error in the billing office or possibly by the physician or person filling out the billing slip—two check marks instead of one. The error was discovered because I called the insurance company to see why they had not paid the bill. When they explained, I called the provider and relayed the information. The charges were immediately reversed. All that to say, don't automatically pay a bill that seems unusual. Twenty minutes on the phone saved us $125.00. Certainly time well spent.

Deductibles and Co-pays

Typically, insurance policies have two different amounts that require out-of-pocket payments by the insured.

Deductibles

Deductibles are the amount that you are required to pay before your policy begins to cover a bill. These vary from policy to policy, so it is wise to find out this information to minimize surprises. Sometimes it will be a flat amount that applies to all bills. An example would be that you are required to pay the first $500.00 of all medical bills no matter where or what. This may apply to each individual in a family or may apply to all members of the family combined.

Sometimes deductibles apply to each separate incidence or procedure. An example of this would be that a policy pays a certain amount for an X-ray and if the charges are more you must pay the rest.

Some insurance companies are contracted with providers and the providers are required to accept their predetermined reimbursement amount and agree to "write-off" and not bill you for the balance.

Deductibles are sometimes determined by you at the beginning of each insurance year; the higher the deductible, the lower your premium. If you are facing a long-term illness and have a high deductible, it might be wise to reevaluate that before the new year begins. You may pay a higher monthly premium to have the lower deductible, but it may be to your advantage in the long run.

Note: Not all insurance companies allow you to change once you are diagnosed. You will need to talk to your insurance provider regarding their policy.

Co-Pays and Other Out-of-Pocket Expenses

After you have met the deductible amount on your insurance, most policies will then pay a percentage of the balance. Seventy or eighty percent is usual. You may be required to use in-network providers. Be sure to check before you begin.

- Copays for office visits that remain consistent throughout the year (and have no deductible)
- Penalties for using out-of-network providers
- Non-covered services

Be aware that insurance deductibles start over every year. This may be at the calendar year, i.e., January 1, or at another predetermined date. Medicare deductibles start over on January first. Many private policies begin on the date that you took it out. Policies with companies where you are employed usually start over on a date determined by the company. When the policy year starts over each year, you will be required to again meet all deductibles and co-insurance.

If you have Medicare, you may also choose to carry a Medicare supplement policy. These policies typically cover the amounts not paid by Medicare. These policies can be confusing. They are offered by many providers. No matter who you purchase your policy from, however, the options are consistent. You will be asked to choose between a number of different plans—these plans are titled Plan A, Plan B, etc. No matter what company you purchase it from, Plan A for example, by law must provide the same coverage as Plan A from any other company. Your cost might be different between companies. This is the reason that you should shop around. Look at your *Medicare & You* booklet. Look at the section on Medicare Health Care Choices and determine which plan is best for you. Then shop for the company that can provide that plan for the lowest price. You have the option to make a change in your insurance providers each year, usually in November or December.

Know your insurance policy/policies. If you have more than one insurance policy, be certain that the bill has been submitted to all companies before you write a check to pay the balance. My sister, who handles insurance claims every day, advises, "When you receive a statement in the mail from your insurance company, read it carefully. If the total amount of the bill has not been paid, check further to see if it has been sent to secondary providers." Insurance is an ever changing business. Do not assume that what was covered last year is covered this year. Know your policy. If you don't understand it, call the insurance company. They have customer service personnel whose job it is to explain it to you. Be sure that you ask for detail. For example, do not just ask "Does my policy cover this?" but ask also, are there deductibles, copay, or non-covered services?"

Example: Your policy has a deductible of $500.00 and 80/20 copay up to $2,000.00.

You have a surgery bill for $3,500.00

- You will pay the $500.00 deductible
- You will pay 20% of the remaining $1,500 of the copay = $300.00

Your total payment due on this bill is
$500.00 + $300.00 = $800.00

- Insurance will pay 80% of $1,500.00 = $1,200.00
- Insurance will pay 100% of the amount over $2,000.00 = $1,500.00

Insurance will pay a total on this bill of
$1,200.00 + $1,500.00 = $2,700.00

At this point you have met your deductible and copay for the year so the next bill should be fully covered, except for non-covered items.

Specialized Policies

You may recall that in chapter one, I suggested buying a cancer policy before you saw the doctor. I am familiar with AFLAC and it certainly is a well-advertised and publicized company, but there are many others, so shop around for the one that works best for you.

Policies such as these do not function as health insurance; instead, though they pay on medical activities, the proceeds come directly to you and not to your hospital or doctor. They are meant to help with the many peripheral expenses connected with an illness.

Usually the policy has a flat amount which is paid for the occurrence of a procedure or treatment. Sometimes it is a one-time payment, such

Is it a Waltz or a Jitterbug?

The progression of cancer treatment can take several courses, but the progression is always toward a cure. My pastor wisely says, "God always cures; sometimes on this side and sometimes on the other." For me it was here, on earth. For my husband it was in heaven, where I believe the Bible ensures me he is wonderfully well and gloriously happy.

Cancer treatment isn't always the same. It varies in length, in intensity, in outcome, and in the amount of pain and lingering side effects it produces. Several things make the determination, but two stand out. The first is the type of cancer. What it is and where it is has much to do with what happens next. We can't always control that. Good sunscreen, good diet, and good genetics can help but it isn't one hundred percent.

The second is severity. The further advanced the cancer is when it is diagnosed; the less likely the cure and the more intense and extended will be the treatment. Many cancers can be diagnosed early with good regular checkups and screenings. This book, if nothing else, is about encouraging you to take full advantage of healthy living and health screenings.

Cancer treatment always begins with the tests and evaluations necessary to determine the type of cancer and the extent of progression. Once that is done, a treatment plan can be developed and begun.

Sometimes the plan is straightforward; the cancer is a common type and the treatment methods are well defined. If so, you will likely receive clear information with few needs for choices.

Sometimes, the cancer is uncommon, unusual, or not as well researched. Treatment outcomes may not yet be well documented. One of the questions you will want to ask, once diagnosis is complete, is what the treatment options are, what they will entail, and how long you should expect them to be. Those answers vary. For Stage Two Breast Cancer, I knew from the onset I would have six rounds of chemo, a second surgery, and six weeks of radiation, followed by five years of a preventative drug and regular checkups.

For Stage Three Colorectal Cancer, it was not as succinct. Instead, the plan included a defined number of chemotherapy, a defined amount of radiation, and then reevaluation. Further treatment was then planned based on the reevaluation results. There were forks in the road several times. Sometimes the doctors made or recommended the direction, i.e. "these drugs have ceased to work and we need to try these drugs instead," sometimes my husband made the choice, i.e., "I am tired and I need to take a break from treatment for a few weeks." Always it was collaboration between the treatment team, my husband, and me.

The following describes Orin's process. The treatment was well defined; the disease progressed past an easy cure on discovery.

Diagnosed in October: Surgery Number One

Surgery followed just two days after the ominous colonoscopy. With only a slim chance of preventing a colostomy procedure because of the location, the surgeon began. Guided by God's hands, however, the colostomy was avoided and we praised God for this first small victory. Six weeks later, just after Thanksgiving, the chemotherapy began, followed by radiation. We were hopeful. We attended my company Christmas party, enjoyed our family, and waited. But January brought bad news and another surgery.

Metastasis: Surgery Number Two

December, 2007: The cancer has spread to the lungs.

With this new information, acquired in the reevaluation following the first round of chemotherapy, came a major shift in treatment goals. What was once potentially curable becomes a disease with death looming somewhere ahead. Extending the quality of life becomes the focus. I know that, he does not, and we don't discuss it. Sometimes being a nurse is not a blessing.

January, 2007:
There is a bowel obstruction, either from scar tissue or the
radiation.

This diagnosis followed readmission to the hospital for severe abdominal pain and vomiting. There was no clear conclusion as to why it had occurred. Likely it was a scar tissue from the first surgery or from the radiation. Sometimes bodies just heal that way. Nevertheless a second surgery is performed.

I was still working and in the middle of a CPR instructor class an hour away. I juggle between hospital, work, class, and home. The nights are short.

Complications: Surgeries Three and Four

By April there are more problems and he is referred to a surgeon in Joplin, an hour away. Cancer treatment is put on hold while complications from previous surgeries and treatments are treated. Three weeks and two more surgeries later we come home, this time with an ominous prediction that an unreachable mass is suspicious for malignancy and time may be very short. Treatment is formally stopped and hospice comes.

Blessings sometimes come in strange ways. Believing the situation to be grave, the surgeon completes the Social Security Disability paper I ask him to complete with the word "terminal." Reeling from the reality of it, I almost don't even return it to the Social Security office. Still, I do, and fifteen days later the disability was approved.

One true blessing that resulted from the terminal diagnosis was the opening up of communication. Orin moved rapidly to talk heart-to-heart with me, his sons, and his family. We planned his funeral; he chose and asked his pall bearers. Nothing was off limits. In the depths of our grief, those were yet, precious days of sharing.

A Small Reprieve

Somewhere in the middle of August of that year, it becomes apparent that the surgeon's supposition that time was short was wrong. Orin was improving. He was very thin, but better. We were encouraged. Hospice left. He took a break from chemo and we enjoyed life and each other. My days were filled with work as an RN with the developmentally disabled. It was rewarding and challenging.

Although not well enough to return to his former job, this reprieve from the rigors of treatment allowed him to indulge his love of woodworking. His days, though often shortened in length, were filled with work at the church. He built a sound booth, a welcome booth, and added trim to the windows. They were blessed days. And at Christmas of 2006, we surprised him with the bright yellow truck he admired.

It was short lived, however. Within a month, scans again showed growing tumors in the lungs; chemo resumed. Once again we cycled through chemo, followed by fatigue, loss of appetite, inability to touch anything cold, daily injections to boost his immune system, then better days, and good days, only to be followed by chemo and the return of symptoms.

Periodically, chemo would stop and tests would help the doctors determine its effectiveness. Finally, we went from first line drugs to second line, as his body became immune to the drugs known to be most effective. We again began to see decline.

In the Roller Coaster at the Top of the Hill

In January, two years after the original diagnosis, Orin complained of dizziness. We were thinking it was probably due to weakness, but just to be safe, the doctor ordered a brain scan. Orin drove himself to that appointment. It was the last time he would be behind the wheel. The appointment was at four in the afternoon. When I arrived home from work at five-thirty, it was to a very somber husband.

"Call the doctor," he said. "You have to go back to the pharmacy for medication. The radiologist at the hospital has already called me with the results of the scan and there is a tumor in my brain."

Though we didn't know it at the time, we, like a roller coaster poised at the top of a very steep hill, were in for a frightening downhill plunge.

The medication prescribed was dexamethasone, a steroid. He started it immediately to reduce swelling and prevent seizures. Though other medications would be added, this was the drug that changed everything. (See effects of steroid treatment below.)

Two treatments were ordered for the tumors found in the brain: one was the steroid, used to keep the swelling down around the tumors before and during radiation, and the second was the radiation, a side effect of which would be hair loss.

We had not had a family portrait done for quite a while and decided that now was the time. It was arranged quickly and the day arrived. Our grandson Blake, a shy six, rebelled at the idea of being photographed. My encouragement to him resulted in yet another treasured "story." I told him we must do this family picture now because grandpa was going to lose his hair. Satisfied with that answer, he participated. When finally we were done with the sitting, I noticed Blake, anxiously watching his grandpa. Finally he came to me and whispered, "Is grandpa's hair going to fall out now?"

Normally, when treatment is done, the steroid is slowly decreased and discontinued, with minimal side effects. Sometimes this doesn't work, and in our case it didn't. Each attempt to decrease the medication resulted in disorientation and dizziness. Over time the dose had to be maintained and slowly increased. By March, his muscles were so weak that he could no longer stand up without help, and he was losing the use of his left arm.

And then there was the sugar. Dexamethasone makes you hungry. It makes you crave sugar. Sugar is the worst food you can eat if you have cancer, but we had progressed to comfort not treatment.

On one occasion, while he was still able to get out, my husband asked our son Mike to take him to a local grocery store.

On return I remember saying to Mike, "Well, did you get everything?"

His response explained in a nutshell the effects of the steroid on appetite. He said, "We sure did! Twelve bags of sugar and a loaf of bread!"

He carried in the sacks full of Twinkies, M&Ms, Hershey Bars, cookies, Ding Dongs, Snickers, ice cream, and Oreos. One favorite treat, however, didn't come from the grocery store but from good friends, Donovan and Kathy. Root Beer Barrels (hard sugar candy) were obtained out of town and lovingly transported to his chair side table. I rarely see Donovan and his wife Kathy that I don't think of those precious deliveries and the cheer they brought to us.

Decline was rapid. By May we stopped treatment and resumed hospice care. We purchased a scooter as walking was now impossible. We made a last trip home to his great-nephew's graduation party. Though it was three hours away, we made it a one-day trip. The boys loaded the scooter and their dad into the yellow pickup and I drove. When we arrived, Orin's brothers met us and helped him out. It was a cherished afternoon; a last, and somehow we knew it. When the day ended, his brothers helped him back into the pickup and we returned home, where his sons waited to help us back into the house.

On July first of 2007, we had our last outing—attending the funeral of a beloved lady at our church. Arriving home, our son struggled to help his dad out of the car and into the house. When he was all settled, he said, "Dad, I nearly dropped you. I don't think we should do this anymore."

Very soon we added a hospital bed and a Hoyer Lift. Blessed by an employer who cared and understood, I spent less and less time at work, going only when someone could be here at home with Orin. Those who pitched in were his sister, his niece, my mom, our boys, and several friends, one of whom drove sixty miles just to spend the day.

On July 31, 2007 at one-thirty in the morning, I woke to screams. Orin was in pain and somewhat disoriented. Several hours later after finally calling the hospice nurse to help, we were able to control the pain and things settled. By morning I called his sister and our sons. Sometime in the early evening he slipped into that state that is somewhere between here and beyond. At eleven thirty-nine he slipped quietly into the presence of Jesus. Quiet here, that is; I have no doubts that shouts of joy erupted on the other side.

Dexamethasone Side Effects

Used to decrease inflammation and swelling in his brain, dexamethasone was a necessary drug for Orin. Still, it had serious side effects. Those that affected us most were:

- Sleep Problems—Sleep was difficult. As the dosage increased, the problem became worse. In my own treatment, I experienced the same thing. I did not have to take the medication all the time, but was given it pre-chemo to reduce nausea. I often was up very late that night, if I slept at all.
- Changes in the Shape or Location of Body Fat—Coupled with increased appetite and craving for sweets, Orin weighed well over 200 pounds and his face was moon shaped when he passed away. This was somewhat difficult for people, especially those who saw him infrequently, as the changes were quick and dramatic.
- Muscle Weakness—Effecting large muscle mass, dexamethasone causes progressive weakness. Within three months of beginning the medication, we acquired a lift chair as Orin did not have the strength to stand on his own. Soon, we got a scooter as he became unable to walk. In just a few more weeks, mobility was possible only with the use of a Hoyer Lift. This is a device used to lift and transfer a person using a sling like canvas sheet attached to a large metal frame. Without it, Orin would have been confined to bed.

Other side effects occur with the use of dexamethasone long term, and they can be found at the following website: http://www.drugs.com/sfx/decadron-side-effects.html. The side effects listed above, however, were the ones that most effected Orin.

Mobility Issues

Mobility almost always becomes a problem with a lengthy illness. Weakness and paralysis often are the main culprits. We found that several things made coping easier.

Furniture arrangement can sometimes make mobility difficult. This is not the time to worry about having a show place. Move items that block access to places your loved one needs to go. If you have area rugs or throw rugs, roll them up and store them in the garage. They impede wheelchairs and walkers and can cause falls. Put as large an end table as possible by the chair where your loved one sits. Use baskets or other storage containers to hold the many things they may want access to.

There was a time when my husband was well enough to stay alone, but yet was immobile. We managed by creating quite a stash of items, including snacks that he could easily reach. Always this should include a phone, preferably with a preprogrammed number to someone close by who could come if needed. I am thankful for those who helped during those days, by stopping by to visit and to refill his water glass.

Hospice will not pay for a scooter. If you suspect that one will be needed, secure it prior to initiating hospice services. With a scooter you should also consider the addition of an outside ramp. Our sons built this, but you can also purchase, and in some areas rent a portable one.

Helping Hands

Hands to help are everywhere; you need only to ask. Grateful that we could spend our last days together in our own home, we reached out numerous times. In the morning and evening, one of our sons would come and help with getting up and to the chair, then back to bed; as Orin got weaker those trips increased to several times a day because of his need to rest.

We reached out to others too; neighbors came when I couldn't scoot him up in bed, or when he slipped out of my arms and to the floor as we tried to maneuver on our own. Once in the night, when all others were sleeping, our local police slipped in and helped.

Our son, Mike, reminds me, "People want to help, but don't know what to do." Mike says, "Tell people they just need to ask."

Survival Tips

- Ask for help.
- Rest when you can.
- Talk and reminisce with your loved one; enjoy each moment.

What a Friend Can Do to Help

- Stop by frequently, but don't stay long unless you are needed.
- Send a note if you can't stop by. It will be appreciated. I had one dear friend that sent a note nearly every week. It was such a blessing to know she was thinking of and praying for us. Thank you, Lea.
- To men: If the person who is sick is a man, they need you to visit. Please do. I cherish the memory of the several men who came by regularly to sit for a spell and visit with Orin. It was a wonderful break for him and for me too. While they discussed the weather and how the repairs were going on the local road project, I could take a break and focus on an outside task I needed to do.

Points to Ponder

> *He shall cover thee with his feathers, and under his wings shalt thou trust: his truth shall be thy shield and buckler. Thou shalt not be afraid for the terror by night; nor for the arrow that flieth by day; Nor for the pestilence that walketh in darkness; nor for the destruction that wasteth at noonday.*
>
> **—Psalms 91:4–6**

> *When thou passest through the waters, I will be with thee; and through the rivers, they shall not overflow thee: when*

thou walkest through the fire, thou shalt not be burned;
neither shall the flame kindle upon thee.

—Isaiah 43:2

Both of these verses from God's Word tell us that He is here, with us, around us, leading and protecting us. We don't always remember. We don't always trust. Just for today, practice leaning on Him for every need. Ask Him to direct your thoughts and steps. Make a decision to believe that He will.

Chapter Seven

Changing Roles

. . . .

Driving somewhere in the middle of the Arkansas hills I said to him, "Where do we turn?"

My former truck driver, always-aware-of-navigating-the-highways husband said, "I don't know where we are."

I knew that for the first time in forty-three years I was in charge of the road.

. . . .

It matters little what your relationship was before. What matters now is you realize change will happen. Don't fear it. If it was great before, it may now be different, but it may be even better. If it wasn't so great, well, many times I have seen God use such a situation to provide an opportunity for greatness to happen. There is something about the frailty of illness and the necessity of human needs that breaks down the barriers that may have kept you apart.

Male or female, as the caregiver you may now find you have become the decision maker, bill payer, cook, nurse, driver, housekeeper, appointment scheduler, and on and on. This can be overwhelming as you try to balance roles you have never had with those already keeping your day full. Examining your priorities, prayer, and the humility to allow others to help can go a long way in easing your burden. Remembering that this is also difficult for the person who is ill can also help you to not become grouchy or short tempered when you are tired, lonely, or scared.

Emotional Responses to Role Changes

Our emotional responses to changing roles can be triggered by a sense of loss. We may already know we are grieving but don't realize how the changes that are occurring affect us.

Grief is about loss. Losses happen every day: quiet time in the morning cut short because we overslept and now we are late; losing our turn in the checkout line because we decided to go back for another item; missing the praise we hoped to get but don't because our grade on the final was a B—not the coveted A+. Most times we lose, grieve, and move on without even a thought. It may not even occur to us that how we react at any given moment may be related to the grief. Different stages of grief cause different reactions. Here are some examples of how this might play out. When you have read these, stop and reflect on your own situation. You may be able to understand some of your own reactions. Knowing is a step to moving on.

Example

John and Mary were normally happy and easy going; both carried their own weight when it came to household tasks. Now, however, John is seriously ill and Mary is now responsible for the tasks of both. Where they are in moving through the grief stages, will affect how they respond to the task of the moment. This time, the furnace filter needs changed.

Mary, the caregiver, might respond in one of the following ways:

- Denial thinks: It really won't matter if they are changed, my electric bill will still be high.
- Anger thinks: I can't believe he expects me to do that; it's not my job!
- Bargaining thinks: If I change the filters myself, maybe he will feel better.
- Depression thinks: I can't deal with that today; I'm too overwhelmed.
- Acceptance says: "The filters need changed. I need you to teach me how to do that."

John, the patient, responds with:

- Denial thinks: The furnace filters need changed; I'll do it when I am better.
- Anger says: "The furnace filters need changed. What's the big deal? Just do it."
- Bargaining thinks: Lord, if you will just let me feel good enough to change those filters, I won't ever complain again.
- Depression thinks: I'm worthless. I can't do anything anymore. I might as well die.
- Acceptance says: "Honey, I usually change the furnace filters every month. You might have to do it this time. When you have time, I will tell you how."

It can be very challenging to not take personally what the other person says, especially if they are angry. Pay attention to what you each are saying and realize that it isn't about you—either of you. This is not a walk for sissies. The hill will be easier to climb if you hold hands.

But I've Never Done That Before

Many years ago we were friends with a retired couple living near us. They lived by the now nearly extinct traditional roles. Each had their duties dictated by 1940s standards of who did what and when. Every day they ate a big breakfast in the morning and a big meal at four in the afternoon. Every meal was prepared entirely by the wife. I never knew Ed to set foot in the kitchen except to eat.

One day, the wife got sick. It wasn't a long illness, and soon, Ed was a widower. Soon after the funeral, he did something I have never forgotten. Ed asked for help from a nephew who was a good cook. Each day for several weeks, this nephew, at Ed's request, came to his house, and step by step, taught Ed to cook.

I was a young bride at that time, but many years later, as a widow, I used that lesson to help me move into the role of living alone. You can too.

Organizing Your Finances

In my experience, it seems that in most families, there is one who is the financial manager and one who doesn't have a clue. How being suddenly left with the financial decisions affects you will depend on which one you are. In either case, some things will change. The first is income. It may lessen or increase, but it will change. Things that will affect this are:

- Job Benefits—Does the person have benefits that continue in the face of illness or long-term disability? If so, how will those change at death?
- Insurance—Does the person have a disability policy, and if so, how long does it last? In our case, my husband had a disability policy that lasted a little over a year. It ceased about the time that he became eligible for social security disability. I marveled at God's goodness and timing for providing for our needs. Incidentally, do not overlook benefits that may be in place with loans or credit cards. Some will make the

payment or even pay the balance if you are disabled or unable to work.

- Life Insurance, Pensions, and Retirement Funds—While these may not come into play while your loved one is still alive, it is well to examine them now. Be sure, among other things, they are all properly and legally correct. Check that beneficiaries are correct and present. Even though we thought we had done all of this, I discovered much later that one fund had no beneficiaries listed. It required a death certificate and a statement that required legal assistance to correct.

- Social Security or Disability Benefit—If your loved one is receiving these benefits, be aware that they must be alive the entire month to receive the benefit. In our situation, my husband died on July 31 at 11:39 PM. The entire July benefit had to be returned.

- Property, Bank Accounts, and Ownership Issues—If it is possible, now is a good time to look at all those situations where your loved one's signature may be required. Bank accounts, property owned, especially those with titles, loans, or other items requiring signatures for transactions to occur, should if necessary be changed now, while your loved one is able to sign what is needed. It would be wise to consult your bank, any insurance or other agents you work with, your attorney, etc., regarding any changes needed. It is not necessary that your loved one's name be removed from the accounts, rather that the participants be listed in such a way as to allow you to transact any business or changes without their approval or signature.

Power of Attorney, Living Wills, Wills, and Wishes

If you have not already done so, now is the time to consider your loved one's wish regarding the last stages of his/her life. They may not be able to tell you when the time comes, so as difficult as the conversation may be, it is one you should have beforehand. There are several documents that you could need and should consider putting into place.

- A medical power of attorney allows the designated person to make medical decisions for someone who is no longer able to do so.
- A financial power of attorney allows the designated person to act in financial situations for a person unable to carry out these tasks.
- A living will directs medical personnel in regards to whether CPR or other life prolonging activities are to be done.

Each state may be different in what is required to enact these documents. Your physician or your attorney should be able to help you. The hospital or hospice social worker is also a good source for direction in these matters.

Social Security and Disability

My husband was fifty-nine when he was diagnosed with cancer. When it became apparent that a cure was not likely and that we would eventually lose the battle, several people encouraged us to apply for Social Security Disability. At first we hesitated, but then took the steps to do so.

I look back on the many miracles of God's care during that time. Certainly this was one. Just prior to the application interview, a setback had required hospitalization and surgery. The findings caused the physician to write "terminal" on the required medical statement form that was to be submitted to the Social Security office. Fifteen days later, the disability was approved. While the word was hard to hear and see, it resulted in the financial support that was to get us through the next years and months. This became more and more of a blessing as my work schedule had to be decreased to provide ever increasing care. Once again God provided.

Reviewing your Financial Plan

I have included the following information written by my son, Mike. Hopefully it will either affirm that you are on the right track with your own financial planning in regards to caring for your family in the event of untimely death or illness, or it will stir you to consider what changes you might want to make.

We can't control when we die, but the reality is we will eventually die. What we can control is how we have prepared and how well our loved ones are taken care of when we're gone. I understand that there are a lot of people who don't like to talk about such unpleasant things as death. If you are one of those people, get over it. Life isn't always fun. Many of the medical test we get aren't exactly fun either, but they can save our lives. So if you're still able, make a financial plan and talk to your loved ones about what to do if something unfortunate should happen. If we were to die today, the last thing any of us would want is for our loved ones to worry about finances in addition to mourning our loss.

When we discuss taking care of loved ones, life insurance is a good place to start. How much do you need? As much as you can afford? Absolutely not! You may not need any at all or you may need more than you can afford. For instance, someone who is not married and doesn't have children will need very little. If they have enough money in savings to cover the cost of their funeral, they may not need any at all. On the other hand, someone who is married with several children and a mortgage may need quite a bit. Even if you are not the primary bread winner, it may be a good idea to have some life insurance. As unpleasant as it might be, stop for a minute and think about what it would be like for your spouse if you died today.

In order to assess your needs and determine whether it should be a term or a whole life policy, consider your current situation and how will it change over time. Be honest with yourself; if you are not, you will only hurt your loved ones. If you are not a good money manager and realistically expect to be dependent on yours and your spouse's job income until you retire, then you should consider a whole life policy for each of you. In addition, it may be worth your time to sit down with someone who does have more financial skills and have them help you with this part. However, if you have some other investments in place that will continue to grow (make sure they are diversified) to the point that even before you retire either of you could survive well on your own, then you may only need a term life policy to protect against premature death.

Children are a consideration here too. We want to make sure they are taken care of as well, but as they grow up they will become more self-sufficient and less dependent on you. The combination of children moving out on their own, you paying down current debts, and increasing investments can change your situation to the point that not as much income is needed ten to twenty years from now. Be realistic though; if your finances haven't improved in the last five years, don't expect them to in the next five. And if you're going to err, do so on the side of caution.

Many books have been written on financial planning and there are many skilled people who can help you with this. My goal here is not to tell you how to set up your plan, but rather to give you a very brief introduction to the process and hopefully get you to think about something that far too often gets put off until it is too late. There are so many things that we can't control in this life—this is one that we can and should. Remember, failing to plan and planning to fail more often than not have the same results.

Survival Tips

- Don't be afraid to talk about what is happening. Pretending things haven't changed won't help.
- Choose a time when you are both at a good place emotionally and physically and discuss the practical aspects of what needs

done. Remember, you don't have to make an exhaustive list at the first sitting. Once the topic is not "taboo," you will find it is easier to discuss those things as they come up.

- Be respectful of the other person. Realize if you are the caregiver that the person who is sick is likely feeling guilty about not being able to carry their share of the load. If you are frustrated say so, but don't blame each other. Channel your energy at the problem, not each other.
- Pray. God knows what you need, so ask.
- Don't be afraid to ask for help. If your spouse is still able, ask them to teach you. If not, find a trusted friend, neighbor, or church member to ask.
- Ask specifically for what you need. "Would you be willing to show me how to change the furnace filters?"
- Offer to return the favor. "What can I do to return the favor?" or even better, "I know you both work. I am good at mending and sewing on buttons; do you have things I can fix for you?"
- Read—Use the library or search online. You can find out how to do about anything using these two resources. When you figure out the "how," then you can make an informed decision about whether to tackle it yourself or get help.

What a Friend Can Do to Help

- Imagine yourself in the other person's shoes. What would you want someone to do or say to you?
- Offer to help. Likely you can anticipate things that need done if you think about it. Offer to do those things.
- Don't be afraid to ask. Don't be afraid to talk about the obvious. Use the feel, felt, found guide: i.e., "Last night I was thinking about how you must feel pretty overwhelmed. I was feeling pretty helpless not knowing what to do or say to help. I thought, I just changed my furnace filters and I'll bet that needs done at your house. Would you like me to take care of that for you?"

Understand that either person may respond to you by saying they are fine and don't need help, crying, getting angry, offering to pay you to do the task, or gladly accepting your help. Remember, it's not about you. Allow the person to be, feel, and say what they need to even if it is negative. Once their feelings are expressed, they will probably be relieved and thank you for both your help and your emotional support.

Points to Ponder

> *I can do all things through Christ who strengthens me.*
> **—Philippians 4:13**

Philippians 4:13 is an often quoted and used scripture. It may also be one that is often misused or misunderstood. It does not say or infer, "I can do everything that I want to do through Christ who will give me whatever I want."

He will get you through. That is a certainty. But it's His way and His things and His time. As with other promises in the Bible, it was also not intended for all mankind, rather, was a promise of a loving God to His children. John 3:3 says, "Jesus answered and said unto him, Verily, verily, I say unto thee, Except a man be born again, he cannot see the kingdom of God."

If you have never taken the steps to become a child of God, do it now. Open the door to God's eternal blessing and direction in your life while He is calling. (See *Afterword: What the Bible Says.*)

Chapter Eight

Death Comes Softly

•••••••••••••••••••••••••••••••••

"I'm tired," he said. "I want to go home." And
I knew he meant to Jesus.

•••••••••••••••••••••••••••••••••

Accepting the Inevitable—
Negotiating Your Loved One's Changing Focus

Sometimes slowly and sometimes suddenly your loved one may begin to change his focus. Perhaps this analogy will help. Once there was a worm who wanted to eat an apple. Terminal illness is like the apple. In the beginning the apple is in front of the worm, but if he stops to look around he still sees the tree and the sky. At the end, the worm is inside and all he can see is apple. Do not be offended when your loved one seems to no longer notice things that are going on around them.

I remember the day I realized the things around us no longer mattered to my husband. Where once he would have noticed the yard

79

needed mowed or the plants watered, now there seemed no interest in what was happening outside of his personal space. Even with me he was sometimes distant. One day he told me "I'm tired; I want to go home." And I knew he meant to Jesus.

I still cooked his favorite meals; he still ate them, and in his always gracious way, thanked me for my efforts. Friends still came to visit and they discussed the things that men discuss. There was, however, an underlying tone his thoughts were elsewhere. It made me sad to see him moving into a place where I could not go, a place between here and his home beyond. I cried more then, usually alone, sometimes with friends, and occasionally with him.

This is not a signal to treat your loved one as though he is no longer present or aware. Instead, let it become your passion to spend precious moments together talking about all that matters most. Talk with them, not about them. If it is necessary for you to talk about what is happening and you may well need to, do so well out of your loved one's hearing. This may be a good time to take advantage of an offer to just get away and go for a soda. You too can become like the worm, so deep inside what is happening that you lose your perspective.

Moving from Active Treatment to Hospice

The day will come when your loved one will decide that treatment needs to be over. In most cases, unless incapacitated and unaware, that decision it theirs not yours to make. I remember that day too. He just simply said, "I'm done. I don't want to take the chemo anymore."

I still struggle some when I remember my emotions that day. Mostly, I remember feeling relief. Cancer treatment is hard work. The endless cycles of doctor's visits, chemo treatment days, feeling sick, waiting for test results—it's a lot. And it's even more in the face of the certain knowledge that one day, the battle will be lost. The decision to stop meant, for the moment at least, that we could just rest and be. And it moved us into a new world that was all about comfort and peace and loving each other.

Help from Hospice

Occasionally I hear someone say, "That's the best invention since sliced bread." That's how I feel about hospice. I encourage you to involve them early in your treatment and care planning, even if they don't actively begin. I am sad when I hear that someone waited until the last few days to utilize their services.

I have had others close to me who have not had such a good experience with hospice care, and I have included information to help you assess and get the care you need. My daughter-in-law recently shared with me her frustrations with the hospice that provided care for her father. One thing she said to me is especially worthwhile in passing on to you. When you assume the caregiver role, you must realize that you have now accepted responsibility for your loved one's needs. You cannot be bashful about advocating to get needs met. You do not need to be unkind, not ever, but you will have to be clear, direct, and ask for what you need.

As an RN, I am very good at advocating for what a patient needs. My personality helps, and I have had a lot of experience at it. It was very easy for me to stay on top of the care and the care items that were needed. It was not difficult for me to ask for a change in a care provider on one occasion, when I felt it was in my husband's best interest.

This is not always the situation, however, and the tasks and decisions you face may seem overwhelming. Do not be timid about asking to visit with the social worker. If you have a friend who has knowledge and skill in this area, tell them how you feel and let them help you.

Here are some things you should consider when choosing a hospice provider. It will be important to know what the hospice will provide to you, as not all provide the same things. Ask about the size of the hospice, how long they have been in business, and whether they are privately owned or a nonprofit organization. What is their experience? Ask for references.

Typically an RN will supervise your care and is the liaison with the physician. You may see them infrequently in the beginning, and daily toward the end. It will be up to you to let your RN know when she is needed. Do not hesitate to call.

It may be important to ask about the experience and back up of the RN who will be providing care. Most hospice nurses are experienced, caring individuals. What you want to know is, what happens if my nurse is less experienced or less caring, does she have back up? Do I have someone to call if I am not satisfied with the care we are receiving?

You may want to ask how far the nurses who will see you live from you. Hospices may have their offices in one county but employ nurses in several. Where the office is doesn't matter much, but if your nurse lives two counties away, it will be less likely that she can get to you quickly if needed. Ask also about how much area the nurses cover. You will want to inquire especially about after hours and weekends. If one nurse is on call with no backup and covers several counties, she may not be available when you need her to come. While it is always possible for a situation to occur when a delay might happen, it is much more likely if she is expected to cover too wide an area and client load.

Ask what medications and supplies are provided. I would ask about the current medications your loved one is taking, any restrictions on what is provided, and the length of time it takes to get refills or new medications if ordered. You want to know that medications needed quickly can and will arrive without delay. Ask about supplies. I have included a list of supplies for your reference. You may not need all of them, but you should know from the beginning which ones they will provide when needed and how long it will take them to arrive. Do not hesitate to ask for what you need. If a supply is becoming low, call ahead so it can be brought to you on the next visit.

Supply Check List (All of these may not be provided. Know before you begin.)

- Hospital bed
- Wheelchair
- Commode
- Bath chair
- Walker
- Cane
- Hoyer Lift
- Scooter

- Lift chair
- Catheter supplies
- Colostomy supplies
- Oxygen concentrator
- Portable oxygen
- Oxygen tubing and supplies
- Breathing machines and supplies
- Latex or vinyl gloves
- Lotions
- Wipes
- Bed pads, bed pan, and urinal
- Bandages, tape, and other wound care supplies
- Heel and elbow protectors

In addition to the RN, an LPN and/or care aides will come to provide such services as bathing and dressing changes when those are needed. Do not hesitate to ask for the help you need. One thing to be aware is that some hospices have volunteer staff that will come. They are limited, however, in that they are not allowed to give direct care. They may help you with shopping or other household items, and they can sit with the person, but you must be available if care is needed as they have a no-touch policy.

Once you have discussed the physical care and availability, ask also about the other services and staff. Usually there is a social worker and chaplain who are on staff and will visit you. Sometimes counseling for family and a support group is available. Again, do not hesitate to ask them to explain what services they do and do not provide.

Moving to hospice should happen when active treatment ceases. As with home health, a doctor's order is needed. You will have the opportunity to discuss all that has happened, all that is going to happen, and all the things you need in the process. Hospice is a total package. Once initiated and in place, you will, for the most part, no longer have to concern yourself with doctor's visits, getting medication, or treatment supplies. This works best when there are no surprises and you have taken the time beforehand to find out about the provider you chose.

The hospice nurse will be your "go to" person, and she or one of her fellow team members will be available twenty-four hours a day, seven days a week. In our situation, the hospice provided the hospital bed, commode, walker, wheelchair, Hoyer Lift, all medications needed for comfort care, and all supplies needed for wound care. They even assumed responsibility for things that we previously needed, such as colostomy supplies. They did not provide medications for conditions not related to the cancer or comfort care. I believe that we may have had one or two such medications, but otherwise all was covered. Our nurse communicated with the physician and on more than one occasion showed up after hours to meet our needs.

The nurse came weekly in the beginning. As the days progressed, the nurse's visits were almost daily. Since there is a nurse on call twenty-four hours a day, seven days a week, a hospice nurse was with us for nearly the entire twenty-four hours before Orin died. This isn't always possible, but we were blessed by her presence and help.

A hospice aide came twice weekly to provide help with baths and physical care. If needed two would come together. They provided much needed help and a bit of respite for me. Take advantage of their presence to move away physically and mentally, and rest for a few minutes.

There was one thing that hospice did not provide. In the end, my husband could not walk and needed a mobile scooter. Somehow it didn't fall into the category of covered items. Before moving from regular care to hospice, we should have gotten that. My advice is to talk to your doctor before you make the switch, and try to anticipate items or things that might be needed but are not covered.

The Payment Changes with Hospice Care

When you move from treatment-focused medical care to hospice care, it is a complete change in what and how things are paid for. Hospice care providers receive a flat daily rate and are expected to provide all items including hardware such as beds and commodes, supplies such as bandages, and any medications that have to do with providing comfort or treating symptoms or side effects of the illness. The daily reimbursement covers the nursing and nurse aide care that you will need. It also includes visits from the chaplain and social worker. Together they should be able to meet the needs that you have or find resources to do so.

What to Expect in the Last Days of a Terminal Illness

There are some things that commonly occur at the last stages of life. The following is a summary of facts found at http://www.Cancer.gov/cancertopics/factsheet/Support/end-of-life-care.

End of Life Signs

Withdrawal from friends and family:

It is common, as death nears, for the person to lose interest in their surroundings and become more internally focused. "Things" in their surroundings are just not important any more. I choose to see this as God's way of drawing the person closer to Himself as He prepares for the time when He will finally transport Him home.

Sleep changes:

Sleep may increase as the person becomes more ill. He or she may even begin to be less aware of surroundings and people. Alternately the person may become more restless, with sleep interruptions and signs of anxiety or worry. It is important to continue to talk to the person as though they are hearing what you are saying, even if you are not sure. Never talk about the person in their hearing or presence even if they appear completely comatose and unaware.

Hard-to-control pain:

Pain may become more difficult to control and may require increases or changes in medication. Your hospice nurse is a specialist in pain control and should be used whenever needed. Do not worry or concern yourself with the possibility of addiction to a narcotic pain substance. It just isn't an issue. Do be aware that increases of medication can cause an increased risk of harm from fall or other injuries, so leaving the person unattended may not be wise.

Increasing weakness:

Weakness and fatigue will increase as the illness progresses and the approaching death gets nearer. It becomes progressively important to arrange activities so that energy is conserved and used for important activities.

Appetite changes:

A decrease in appetite is common. The body's need changes as does its ability to use and process food and drink. We experienced something different. Seven months prior to my husband's death, he was diagnosed with metastasis to the brain. A steroid was added to his medication regimen to treat swelling and prevent seizures. Steroids make you hungry. He ate well and craved sugar to the very end. This is not the usual course, however. The cessation of intake of food and liquids often signals that the end is but a few days away.

Awareness:

On occasion they may report seeing or speaking with loved ones who have already died. They may report seeing Jesus or a bright light. They may talk about going on a trip. Unless the person seems disturbed, it's okay to ask them to say more about what they see or hear. Do not tell them that what they are seeing or hearing is not there or discount the reality of what they say. Remember that we are flesh and blood, but we live in a spiritual world. God uses many ways to encourage and comfort His children. Psalm 116:15 tells us, "Precious in the sight of the LORD is the death of his saints." Those who are Christians know and believe that the Word of God is truth. If we are so precious to Him that He thought to include a confirmation of it in His Word, is it not likely He would be very near and very comforting as we anticipate our coming to Him?

Near the end of life confusion may occur. There are several reasons for this. Decreases in food and fluid intake may result in electrolyte imbalances in the body and confusion is a direct result of this. Sometimes this is related to the need to increase medications to control pain.

Another cause of confusion may be the growth of tumors in the brain. This can be expected if brain metastasis is known. It may also be a signal that this has occurred even if a formal diagnosis has not been made.

As death nears, the person will in many cases be less alert, and eventually may be comatose. This may happen in a short period of time, but especially with long and progressive illnesses, may happen more slowly over a period of days. The cessation of intake of food or water is an indicator that this may be nearing.

Changes in body functions:

Because food and fluid intake is decreasing there is likely to be a decrease in bodily secretions. Organs are beginning to slow or stop. Urine becomes concentrated and therefore will appear dark in color. Bowel functioning may cease, or conversely move without control. The important thing now is comfort. Deal with what is. Disposable pads will or can be provided by hospice. Keep them dry and clean. Be aware that perspiration may also result in a need to change the pads.

Lotion, powder, gentle massages, and backrubs can be soothing to the person. They are also an important way for you to help, have contact, touch, and sooth. It can be an important part of letting go. Soon your loved one will be leaving the physical world and touch will not be available. Savor the contact now while you can. Know that each moment is precious. Say what you have needed to say. Do not be shy about it, and don't hesitate to ask others to leave you alone if you wish privacy. They will understand.

Breathing:

As death nears, breathing patterns may change. It may become irregular. There may be periodic moments when it seems as if the person is holding his breath. Long pauses may frighten you, but they are part of the process. If gurgling sounds occur, it is because fluids and saliva have collected in the back of the throat. You may turn the person on their side if you wish. Normally this is not causing your loved one distress, however; it is just part of the process. If you begin to notice changes in breathing and your hospice nurse is not present, it would be good to let them know of the changes. They will likely come if at all possible and this will be comforting and helpful to you.

Skin changes:

As circulation decreases you will likely notice that the skin becomes paler, even bluish in color. Mottling may occur, especially on the legs and feet and may progress as death nears. Mottling, the result of the decreased blood flow, looks like patches of dark, light, and even reddish spots. Nothing needs to be done. Your loved one is not in pain because of it. Do not treat is as if the person is cold. Never use electric blankets or heating pads as this may cause burns. A light blanket is all that is necessary if your room is of a normal comfortable temperature. Do report skin changes to the nurse if she is not aware of it.

Death

This is a difficult section to write because there is no one description of what that moment will be like. In many cases, the person slips deeper into unawareness and it almost seems as if they are truly gone before their body quits working. If you have not experienced it, that may be hard to understand. My husband left that way. The last hours that he was alive, he seemed deeply asleep and unresponsive to our words or touch. His breathing was somewhat irregular, and his heartbeat was fast. When his body finally stopped and it was over, I felt a bit like I do on New Year's Eve when I wait and wait for midnight to come, and when it finally arrives, nothing happens. He had been gone from me for several hours. His body stopping was only the ending of his earthly functioning.

My dear grandmother and mother-in-law both sat up and were able to eat not long before they died. Their passing was peaceful and uneventful, almost as if they fell asleep.

I have witnessed on several occasions, death that was a struggle. A friend took off her oxygen at the end, refusing to allow it to be put back. She was a Christian; she knew where she was going, and was anxious for peace with her savior. Her body, however, already reacting from the low oxygen levels struggled. It was hard for all of us, although I again felt that she had already gone home and we were really just witnessing her body's last involuntary reactions.

Death may be so sudden that there is no anticipation, no preparation, and no awareness of its coming. My daddy hadn't felt well and he and mom had stayed home from church that Sunday morning. He got up about ten o'clock, told my mom he felt better, and had even gotten dressed. Now in my house growing up, if you had been sick, your first meal was always a poached egg. Mom asked him if he wanted one, moved to the stove to cook it, heard a thud, and when she turned he was on the floor, already gone.

As a nurse, I witnessed many who just seem to fall asleep and slip into eternity. I witnessed those who struggled and those who just seemed unable to let go. I don't know why it's not always the same. I do know that God does. When we are His, leaving our earthly home means arriving at our new home with Him. I think however it happens, the trip must be glorious!

How Do You Know that Death has Come?

Sometimes it can be difficult to know, especially if breathing has become irregular, slower, and the person is unresponsive to touch or sound. However:

- Breathing will cease. It is not uncommon for there to be a last gasp or two even after you believe that the person is not breathing any longer. This is simply a reaction as muscle functioning stops and relaxation happens. It is not uncomfortable for the person at all.

- There will be no pulse. Pulses may be found in the wrist just down from the thumb, and in the neck below the jaw bone. As death approaches, pulses may become weaker and faster. This is a result of lower blood volume circulating in the person's body. Unless an IV is kept in place to infuse fluids, this happens naturally because the person has not been eating or drinking normally.

- Eye movement stops. Blinking stops. The pupils of the eyes are enlarged. Eyelids may be open or closed.
- The jaw and face will relax.
- The body may release bowel and bladder contents.
- The skin becomes pale and cool to touch.

It is helpful if there is a hospice nurse there with you. They will take care of everything that needs to be done. If they are not, but you have hospice in place, call them. If you do not and it is unexpected, call 911 and they will respond and help you.

It is best if, as you become aware that the end is near, you have family or a friend stay with you. When death comes, you may do whatever is comfortable for you and your family. Place a pillow under their head; cover them with a light sheet. Spend whatever time you need with the body and your family if they are there. Talk, pray, hold their hand, say goodbye. There is no longer an emergency and you do not need to be rushed in this process. Much of this information, in addition to my own experiences, has been summarized from the National Institute of Health website. Full information may be found at http://www.cancer.gov/cancertopics/factsheet/Support/end-of-life-care.

Sudden Death

"I'm feeling better," he said. Minutes later, my seventy-seven-year-old father collapsed and was gone.

•••••••••••••••••••••••••••••••••••

"I'm going to bring home a pizza for supper," she said.

"Stop and pick up a gallon of milk, we are out," he responded. When she arrived home, my niece found her husband dead, at age fifty.

•••••••••••••••••••••••••••••••••••

Sudden death—unexpected, unannounced, often at too early an age—changes much of what has been said in the previous sections. With chronic illness, plans are made, roles are slowly transferred, and the future considered.

Grief began for me at diagnosis, as I saw our lives plummeting toward change over which I had no control. It intensified three months later with the spread of the cancer signaling unlikely recovery.

Each loss, each change, brought new feelings and emotions.

After my husband's funeral, I stood at one point, talking with someone whose husband had been killed three years earlier in an auto accident, just months before my husband's diagnosis. This woman, a widow, was now three years into the grief process—yet as we talked some things we were feeling seemed nearly identical. It made sense because we essentially had started the grief process at the same time.

Besides the intense and traumatic shock that sudden death leaves in its wake, there are some practical problems that make things very different.

Financial issues will change more drastically when the widow or widower is young. If there is a great insurance policy, the person has a great job, and the kids are receiving Social Security benefits, finances could even improve. This does not, of course, make up for the loss, but it can alleviate at least, this one stressor See *Organizing Your Finances* in Chapter Seven for a more complete discussion of this issue.

Funeral Arrangements

There are many ways to have a funeral. Whatever you choose to do should be for the purpose of the comfort and closure for you and your family. Since the choices of what to do come quickly on the heels of the death of your loved one, thinking about them ahead of time is helpful. You may wish to discuss this with your loved one. Although difficult to initiate, this can be a very sweet time for both of you and it can assure you are doing what will honor them. Do remember, however, that funerals and memorials are for the living. It is you and your family who must find a way to put closure to the death and find a way to move forward.

I felt honored to have the opportunity to discuss and plan for that day with my husband. It again felt as if God had orchestrated the opportunity. About a year into my husband's illness, it was thought that he may have very few months to live. Hearing this prognosis prompted him to have candid conversations with me, his sons, and his friends. We visited the funeral home, planned his service, and picked out a casket, cemetery plots, and stones. He spoke with and asked each of his pallbearers individually. He talked with our pastor. We chose singers. As the day arrived for me to put the final okay on what was planned, there was one song that did not feel right. I desperately wanted a different one, one that spoke to my heart and needs. Wisely, our pastor reminded me that Orin, now in heaven with the Savior, was no longer concerned with this earthly service. I should choose what ministered to me. I did, and have never been sorry. I am quite sure that Orin approved.

Our service was very focused on his life and on his service to God and his family. Salvation and our desire that those who attended know how to attain it was a common goal. Our music was focused on the hope and home of heaven and its glory. It helped me to know that others were hearing about what we as a couple had found. It allowed me, though now alone, to choose to continue in the path we had started together.

This was our ending, but it may not be yours. Not long ago we lost another dear family member. They were horsemen, and had been very involved in a Saddle Club and 4-H. He was young and there was a large circle of friends with similar interests. They wore jeans and boots and cowboy hats. This family chose very differently in how to honor him and find comfort. They chose not a funeral, but a memorial which included western songs they loved, a cowboy's prayer, and a barbeque—absolutely perfect for them.

Choosing no funeral or memorial is also an option that is becoming more popular, as is having a delayed memorial. This is especially true when cremation has been chosen. While I have an opinion about the no funeral option, it is not necessarily wrong. Whatever is done, the important thing is that it allows those who are left behind to grieve and to deal with the death.

My son and his wife have lost both of their fathers to cancer in the last five years. As parents of three young children, they have expressed strong feelings about involving their children in the funeral activities. They chose, in both situations, to use a sitter for the children during the service and visitation. In the first instance, the children were too young to have any understanding of what was occurring. In the second, the children were taken privately to the funeral home, and given plenty of opportunity to ask questions. They were given the opportunity to choose whether to attend the funeral. Mike says, "Only one thing is important, and that is what is best for the child. It should never be about what *looks good* or meets the needs of the adults involved."

Survival Tips

- Pray: Pray now for the calmness and wisdom to deal with the endless pressures of being fully in charge of EVERYTHING … and NOTHING.
- Laugh: Find things to laugh about and, if possible, do it together. We had several experiences that provided laughter, some at the time, and some for later. When cancer begins to interfere with thinking and memory, my husband turned to me in the middle of a visit with family and said "Where is my chocolate bar? I requested it an hour ago!" It was like it came from an unknown sophisticate hiding inside my sweet plain spoken mate. We didn't laugh then, my family and me, and I certainly got that chocolate bar post haste, but now—now it's a sweet memory that brings a smile to an otherwise downcast moment.
- Don't be afraid to talk. Make an effort to think of the things that you may need to know. Reminisce about past experiences and people in your lives.
- Make a daily habit of imagining yourself as the patient instead of the caregiver. How would you want your caregiver to act?
- Quit being a martyr! When someone offers to help, let them.

What a Friend Can Do to Help

- Offer to come and sit with the person while the caregiver runs an errand or takes a break. Say, "I have a free afternoon tomorrow, may I come sit while you do your shopping?" or "I would like very much to spend some time with (name), and I wouldn't mind if you took that as an opportunity to get out and do errands or take a break. When would be a good time?"

- Is there a practical task that needs done? Do it. I saw a perfect example of this not long ago. A friend who quietly without asking cleaned the refrigerator so that it would be ready to receive the many offerings of food that would soon be coming to the door. What a great way to say, "I care."

- Send a memory. My niece, Debbie, says it best in her blog post after Larry's death: "Many of you wrote a note about how you knew Larry, a memory, when you met him or our family, etc. I have decided that I will never send a sympathy card again without including a note of how I knew that person or a memory, because I know these meant so much to me."

Points to Ponder

Let not your heart be troubled: ye believe in God, believe also in me. In my Father's house are many mansions: if it were not so, I would have told you. I go to prepare a place for you. And if I go and prepare a place for you, I will come again, and receive you unto myself; that where I am, there ye may be also.

—John 14:1–3

My husband took great pleasure in building things. He was a perfectionist and what he made was always done quite well. One night after he had gone home, I woke having had a particularly vivid dream of him. He was in heaven, his overalls were pure white, and his hammer hung at his side. He looked happier than I have ever seen him. I was quite assured that he was building mansions and loving every minute. It was yet another assurance to me that I could trust that what God says in His word is true.

....

Part Three

And Then
There Was One

One ring
One call
My heart stops
Driving
Forever
Too late
He is gone
Our sweet daddy
Beloved grandpa
Her husband
She grieves
Move on we say, but she says no
She cannot go
Years pass as grandkids grow and fill her life
Routine becomes her friend
Still she is alone

And then the day
Unspeakable
Cancer
My friend, my love, my life
And he is gone
I cry and scream and say it cannot be
Move on they say
And she says no
Time will pass
Kids will grow
Routine will become your friend
But the hole will always be
I know, I say
Today
My mother is my friend

· ·

Chapter Nine

Alone

···································

It is night again.
I burrow in the downy comforter that has
become my quiet hiding place.
How did I get here?
Why am I alone?
Where are you Lord?
Only yesterday I was hand in hand
with my beloved.
Only yesterday life was rich and full and sweet.
Only yesterday the problems of each moment
were met with anticipation and victory.
Only yesterday.

Death.
When did you come and change my world?
When did you move me from
my lofty perch where all was well?

Propel me down craggy cliffs
that tear at my very being.

Hands.
Steady hands reach out to me.
In the quiet of the night my heart cries
and you pull me close.
I do not know how long we are silent together.
I sleep.

•••••••••••••••••••••••••••••••••••••

Quiet

If it has just been the two of you in your household, you will now be alone. Any noise will come only from you. I found that both comforting and disquieting.

We were blessed to be able to care for Orin at home. I had been the caregiver, but in the last weeks I often had another family member present. Death was going to happen, but I expected that several more weeks would pass before that occurred. I was not prepared for the sudden turn of events on July thirty-first. He woke me that morning at one o'clock, screaming in pain. By noon I sensed the end was near; at 11:39 that night it was over. The next days were a blur of planning and family and friends and food, and then it was over. Hospice came and removed the hospital bed, the lift chair they had loaned us, and the medical supplies; family left, friends went back to work, and suddenly I was alone, all evidences of the past months removed.

The first night alone seemed almost unreal. I remember thinking that it didn't exactly feel as if this was a real situation. Emotions flooded at times and I cried; but those moments were contrasted by numbness. I remember walking around just looking at the pieces of our life together and feeling very, very alone.

Finally, needing to do something, anything, I rearranged the furniture, taking care to put things where they had never been before. I hoped that different would make it better; it just made it seem strange.

The house, our house—my house, was too quiet. Though not much of a television watcher, I turned it on and up. I thought perhaps the noise would be distracting, instead it was irritating. That night I used a sleeping pill. Drifting to sleep, I allowed myself to relax and finally knew the peace of settling into the gentle arms of Jesus.

How soon you return to work is an individual decision. You may need to take a few days or even weeks to rest, recover, grieve, or deal with undone tasks. For me, returning to work seemed right and so I did on the following Monday. I was fortunate enough to have an employer who was wonderfully understanding about my need to be gone while Orin was sick and co-workers who did things to help me keep up. Now, they helped with kind words and hugs, and I found solace in the routine of the job.

Returning home, no matter from where, continued to be difficult for a long time. I steeled myself for entering the door, longing to hear the TV playing, and people talking. On the worst days I found outdoors a better place to be—taking a walk or pulling weeds in the flower bed. They at least seemed to just go on growing as though nothing had changed and somehow that was comforting.

There were also days when I welcomed the quiet. Curled in my favorite chair with a steaming cup of coffee I wrote notes of thank you to those who had meant so much, relished in the comfort of the psalms, remembered, and rested.

Thank You Notes and Dishes

If your loved one was young, or well known, the thank notes that you will want to send will seem overwhelming in number. If that is the case, having someone help you with addressing envelopes can be a good idea. If, however, it is something that you can manage, consider doing it yourself, cherishing each note that you write. I was able to do this and found great comfort in taking the time to remember the relationship we had had with each person or family who had sent their condolences.

It is quite likely that you will also have a few dishes that need to be returned to persons who were thoughtful enough to provide a casserole or pie. What a great opportunity to practice going out on your own. Don't rush; enjoy the visit with each person you see. Consider scheduling to meet them for lunch or coffee. Let returning a dish be the catalyst for starting new habits on your own.

Your Health

Make an appointment with your physicians for a physical. Schedule any screening tests that are due or overdue. Your life has been stressful and you are therefore more prone to disease. Don't wait. Do it now.

Here are a few things you may want to discuss with your doctor:

- Am I due for a mammogram, breast exam, and Pap test?
- Am I due for a prostate exam?
- Am I due for a colonoscopy?
- Will you check my Vitamin D level (new research tells us that deficiencies are more common than once thought)?
- What other things might the stress I have been under affect?

Make a Decision to Trust God with Your Future

Two weeks after my father died suddenly, my mother relates the heart wrenching decision of what to do with my father's cattle herd.

"They were so tame... I talked to the sale barn but they couldn't assure me of what would happen. That night I awoke with nightmares of the calves being separated from their mommas. So I prayed."

The next morning the answer came as her grandson expressed a desire to have his grandfather's herd. "I didn't think I could handle it," she said "but God had it all planned."

I don't know that it is helpful to be told at this point in the journey to "just trust God." Even the most mature of Christians will admit that this is not always an easy task; harder still when your world has just been turned upside down. What I am recommending is that you take a step in that direction. If you are a Christian, make the decision to practice trusting. If you are not, consider becoming one. It is a myth that God's comfort is universally available to all. He desires that, but He requires your trust and faith in Jesus be made before He can truly be all that He desires to be.

A New Relationship

One of the things that was hardest for me was that I finally realized that there was no one who would love me quite like my husband did, and no one that I could talk to who would understand like he did. That is so very hard. Then I discovered that Jesus did and He would. It took time to learn to talk to Him that way and even longer to learn to sit quietly and wait for His response. But He is there and He will know and listen. Learn to even "think" to Him.

Survival Tips

- Relax. It has probably been a while since you have truly done that. I have a porch swing. It's the best ever. I let it be my own little world. A good pillow, a good book, or a good nap. You may not have a porch swing, but find somewhere. I have a friend who lost her husband. She bought a new recliner for her bedroom. One of those big comfy kind. It became her special place. Where ever it is, make it special. Buy a special coffee cup or iced tea glass; whatever it takes to make you feel special.
- Treat yourself to some pampering. Get a manicure, take a bubble bath, and eat ice cream for supper—with chocolate topping.
- Cry when you need to, and then give yourself permission to go on. As hard as it is to live with the pain of loss, sometimes it can be harder to allow yourself to be happy without feeling guilty. It may be necessary to just tell yourself it's okay and do it.
- Find someone you can help.

What a Friend Can Do to Help

- What can you do to help? The answer to this is pretty simple. Help. You now have a family member or friend who is alone. This is what this means. Now there is one income instead of two. There are two hands instead of four. Certainly they don't want or need you to come in and takeover, however, there are likely many things that your friend either doesn't know how to do or is physically incapable of doing. You can be a blessing by sharing their load.

- Be patient.
- It's not always easy to be a friend to the brokenhearted. We can be a time intensive, emotionally draining sort. We don't want to be. We want to be strong. We want to appear as though we are handling things better than anyone else on earth ever has. Usually that isn't what happens and your love and patience will be needed.

Points to Ponder

> *He healeth the broken in heart, and bindeth up their wounds. He telleth the number of the stars; he calleth them all by their names. Great is our Lord, and of great power: his understanding is infinite.*
>
> **—Psalm 147:3–5**

God understands where you are right now. He knows that your heart is hurting and that you are all alone. This is the same God who not only knows every star but knows each by name: how very much more precious are you to Him. He is willing to help you through this valley and He is more than able. Trust Him.

Chapter Ten

Normal Grief

••••••••••••••••••••••••••••••••••

Kubler-Ross stages of grief:

Denial: "This cannot happen to me!"

Anger: "Why did this happen to me? Who's to blame for this?"

Bargaining: "Just let me live 'til my daughter's wedding, and I'll do anything."

Depression: "I am too sad to do anything."

Acceptance: "I'm at peace with what is coming."

••••••••••••••••••••••••••••••••••

Many years ago, during a very difficult time in our marriage and child rearing years (if you are there right now, the answer is stay, it does get better), I attended a workshop given by Elizabeth Kubler-Ross. It made sense to me and has continued to be the framework on which I hang my understanding of what happens in the process of moving from loss to acceptance.

Since then, other descriptions of the process have surfaced. Please know that they are there. If your situation is not fitting my experiences, seek them out. Ultimately it's a road trip and there is more than one route. It is my deepest wish for you to find your path, experience your journey, and emerge with peace and joy in your heart.

No! It can't be!

Denial or Shock

The world is calm and pleasant; or perhaps it's not. Sometimes life is just one crisis after another. Either way, we are always subject to this event. I remember the last huge shock I experienced. We had just started a new piano class. It was a new method that had promise for great results. The lessons required that the child be accompanied by a parent or other adult to act as coach. My son and I decided to enroll his two oldest daughters in the class. We left the first class pleased with our decision and as we drove home, we chatted about our first lesson. We were both looking forward to what we were going to learn and I was enjoying the chance to be part of my granddaughters' experience. It was a great family moment. And then my cell phone rang. It was my sister-in-law with the awful news that her son-in-law, my nephew, had just died of a massive heart attack. It was impossible news.

My husband was the youngest of four children. We were one of those fortunate families that all stayed married and all lived relatively close to one another—we were "a family." We lost my husband at age 65 to cancer, and two or three others of us had some health conditions that could eventually result in an early death. But this was one of the kids and it was sudden. At fifty, Larry was only a few years older than the son who sat beside me in the car. This was not supposed to happen. But it did. For days after, I would shake my head as I tried to process what had happened, trying to believe what I already knew to be true, but could not quite accept.

Anger is like an umbrella, it covers other softer emotions,
such as fear, embarrassment, and hurt; so why am I still mad?

Anger

I remember learning somewhere, many years ago, that anger was not a primary emotion. Instead, it was like an umbrella, covering softer, more vulnerable feelings; feelings like hurt, embarrassment, fear, loneliness. The anger that surfaces with loss is an excellent example of this. It hurts to lose someone you love. Sometimes the intensity it produces explodes in anger and a thousand whys. The following explores some of those feelings in more depth.

Loneliness

Loneliness is very real. In the beginning, it is the loss of just having someone there: waking up to someone on the other side of the bed or having a reason to bake a pie. Later it was the realization that the man who had spent a lifetime learning to know me, love me, and accept me like no one else on earth, was gone. Way before I transferred that to trusting Jesus to meet those needs, I was angry—angry at him, and angry at every other person who attempted to be there for me but fell short because they were not him.

Fear

The realization of all the responsibilities you now have for things you know nothing about results in fear. I felt fear when it occurred to me I could no longer tell him the lawn mower wouldn't start, knowing he would fix it; or when I couldn't remember a name and turned to him to ask—and he wasn't there.

I felt fear when I realized Orin's social security check would be withdrawn from our account. Over the years, I can see how God has taken care of my finances. I don't live in luxury, but the bills get paid. Still, my first reaction was fear that checks would bounce and I would be in poverty. And I was quickly angry—angry at the government over twenty-one minutes and angry at Orin for dying too soon. Later, I was able to turn this into a smile as I remembered he never was the best at managing money. Of course he would die twenty-one minutes too soon. I have found the little things along the way that cause me now to smile are remembrances that keep him very close to my heart, so this one was worth the money.

Embarrassment

Other than too much alcohol, I know of nothing else that results in doing crazy, stupid, and embarrassing things like grief, especially if you are impulsive. People react to loss by getting into relationships too soon, buying houses, expecting the impossible of others, overworking, quitting jobs, overspending, and under eating.

I didn't do all of those, but I did enough to wonder if my credibility as a human being could ever be salvaged. And that made me mad, mostly at myself.

Loss

Somewhere along the line you'll just get angry about what you have lost. This time it isn't even about the person. It's about you, and the things that are no longer part of your world. It may be income, certainly that is a real and tangible item that has a great effect on how you will manage things from here forward, but it is likely much more.

One of the most difficult realizations for me was the awareness that I was no longer part of a couple, and in losing my husband, I had also lost most involvement in social situations where other men were present. It is just awkward. You are a third wheel and the road is built for a bicycle or a car.

"If only we could"

Bargaining

Bargaining is one of our most common tactics to deal with what life gives us. It is most often described in relation to the grieving process as an attempt to justify or blame what has happened on something or someone. Daily, the bargaining process helps us to analyze and make sense of the events that have occurred. If we are lucky we will also learn from them.

"If only I hadn't overslept, I wouldn't have been speeding and gotten that ticket," can result in us buying an alarm clock and changing our behavior. It may not be necessary to remind you that learning doesn't always occur in such situations. Instead, blaming may become a standard response to life's quirks. "Nobody woke me up," or "the traffic was too heavy."

Sometimes bargaining starts way before the death occurs. "God, I'll do anything you ask if you will just let him live."

Why is your world still moving when my world is stopped?

Depression

Depression is a common part of the grieving process. Somewhere past the sadness is the realization that things will never be the same. The time will come when the acute grief is past and others have resumed their lives as though nothing changed. You, alone, know that everything has.

When this occurs, it is not uncommon to get stuck. My best advice to you when that occurs is to just stop. Stop running, stop blaming, stop fixing, and stop trying to get others to understand the pain you are feeling. They don't, can't, and won't. You will need to walk this path alone, unless you know the Lord.

Will I ever stop crying?

When I was in the active stage of caring for my husband, many prayed. When I was too tired or too busy, others bridged the gap. I knew it. I felt it. But the time came when only one thing helped. I stopped. In those dark quiet hours of reflection and tears, the arms of Jesus held me close. Snuggled in the downy comforter on my bed, I felt Jesus's arms and love, and slowly healed.

Is what I am experiencing normal?

These are some of the things that have happened to me or others who I have known personally in the process of grieving.

Tears Happen

We cry when we get hurt. We cry when we are happy. We cry when we are disappointed. We cry when we are sad. Crying is an expected activity with the grieving process. *Tears are good for the soul*, it is said. I believe that is true. There are times when tears can say and release emotions that would otherwise remain stuck in your heart.

Alone is a safe place to cry

Crying in the grieving process can sometimes be a bit different, almost mysterious in its occurrence. Normal "crying" occurs at expected times. I did that too. When someone came to offer comfort; their hug would often trigger tears. Usually though, intense grief surfaced when I was alone.

When I lost my husband, I cried for weeks every time I drove alone in the car. I didn't leave the house crying, I didn't leave church, or the store, or a friend's crying, but the event none the less was consistent and predictable. Somewhere in the space between here and there it would well up in my soul. Tears would sneak out of my eyes, quietly at first, and then almost as if it were a symphony building to a crescendo it would turn to sobs. Soon, anger at my situation spewed out and the sobs turned to screams as my emotions surfaced. I don't know, perhaps I knew that it was safe—alone, driving, unobserved. I would arrive where I was going spent and calm. No one knew about my harrowing trip through the mountains and valleys of sadness, anger, fear, and regret. Well, except God. I always knew He was in the other seat, right there beside me, saying, "Let it out honey, it's okay, and I won't tell."

The first time since

I learned to expect tears, or at least *something* whenever I faced an activity, person, place, or thing that we had previously done together. I think that happens when we are trying to change a habit too. Smokers, once quit, will face triggers that will cause the desire for a cigarette to surface and the first time is always the hardest to overcome.

At first it was constant seeing each friend and family member for the first time since he died. Going into the hardware store where we had purchased supplies for a remodel brought memories long forgotten—and tears. Mowing the yard, the seed catalog that arrived in the mail, the intersection where we had disagreed and argued—each event triggered a memory, and usually a tear. Even now, years later, I will occasionally have a first and it will happen again.

Sometimes for always

There are other things so precious I have learned to expect a tear, or at the very least an awareness and moment of sadness each time they are in front of me. His favorite hymn, walking past the sound booth that he had built in the church auditorium, driving past the Lowe's home center where we always had to go on our periodic shopping trips to Joplin, all continue to be a quick and direct path to the sadness that never quite goes away.

But they never seem to cry

The phrase keeping it *all bottled up inside* is often used to describe someone who just seems unable to express emotions. Certainly this happens. Perhaps men do it more often than women or children. Even today, men are less expected to cry. Perhaps, however, they are just more likely to do it alone—to find expression alone on the freeway or in the harvest field. It is inaccurate to assume that seeing someone in public who appears to be dealing well or handling things does not cry.

Where it is safe

I learned very quickly there were some people who were so uncomfortable with my sadness and tears that I could not, would not, allow my feelings to surface in their presence.

I also learned that this could be a help. Going to church alone was, and remains, difficult. I miss him there more than even at home. I had a few friends at church that seemed to fit in the above category and when I needed or wanted to keep my emotions in check, I could do so more easily by physically putting myself in their close proximity. It never, ever ceases to amaze me, the length that God has gone to in order to provide for our every need.

Sadness

There is a difference between the normal sadness that is experienced in this stage of grief and the dysfunctional depression that we will discuss later. It is normal to be sad; you have lost someone very important. It is not likely that the sadness will ever go completely away, nor is it necessary to. Many years now since my father died so suddenly, I am sad when I remember him and realize that he was taken, too soon from our lives. I am not, however, stopped from life by the sadness. I feel it, and I go forward yet again, with a new resolve to tell my grandchildren stories about their great-grandfather.

Changes in Sleep

Sleep problems are not uncommon. Possibly for many months now you have been sleeping "with one eye open" so to speak; now you do not have to do that. You may find yourself unable to physically go to bed because you are alone. The opposite may be true; you may find that you prefer sleeping to being awake and aware of what has happened. Either way, relax. Some of this is normal and common. If it worsens, does not resolve in a few weeks, or concerns you, see your doctor. He may prescribe a medication temporarily to help get your sleep patterns back in line.

But first, here are a few things to try:

- Milk—Have a glass of milk before bed. Milk has tryptophan in it, a natural relaxant, and when I have had a hectic day, it's the thing that helps.
- A good book—One that will completely distract you can be helpful. If you are like so many of us, a few pages and your eyes begin to get heavy.
- The Good Book—One of my favorite things to do in those minutes before sleep is to review passages of scripture that I

have committed to memory. Or just take one passage or verse and meditate on it. Meditate means to think about it, about what it says, what it means; what God wants you to know from it. Repeat it over and over, slowly focusing on a different word each time:

o   I will never leave you or forsake you
o   I (God, your heavenly Father, Jesus, The Holy Spirit) will never leave you
o   I will (not might, sometimes, if I want to) never leave you
o   I will never (not usually, but always) leave you
o   I will never leave (be absent from, go away, walk off, ignore) you
o   I will never leave you (you means YOU)

- NSAIDS (non-steroidal anti-inflammatory drugs)—I find that I have had a busy day, with lots of physical activities, I may have pain, muscle aches, and such, that aren't really severe but still they leave me just uncomfortable and restless. Acetaminophen, Ibuprofen, or one of the other analgesics can help.

- Over-the-counter sleep medications—Most over-the-counter sleep medications are a combination of an analgesic, like aspirin or acetaminophen or ibuprofen, and diphenhydramine. Diphenhydramine is an antihistamine, used for allergic reactions and sinus concerns, but it has a side effect of sleepiness. Combined with the mild pain relief it can help. Be aware that any of these should not be used on an ongoing basis without your doctor's approval, and of course do not use them if you are allergic to any of the ingredients. Temporarily, however, they may be just the thing to get you past those first difficult nights.

Changes in Eating Habits

I went from cooking three meals a day to two bowls of cereal and a meal at the local café at noon. I still struggle with getting the proper nutrition. It's not much fun to eat alone or cook for one. My hubby was a meat and potatoes man. I could probably be a vegetarian without much effort. He liked spicy things, I like them plain. There are some advantages of cooking just for you. It's like the burger slogan: you can "have it your way." A trip to the local library or bookstore could be a fun way to get out on your own and find new recipes and ideas to fit your new life style.

I did have a few recipes that were some real favorites. It was hard to make them without him there. One was so difficult it even sparked the following poem:

Macaroni and Cheese

Forty two years…a lifetime, since I stood
beside his mother in her kitchen on the farm
until I knew
just how to grate and cut and layer and mix
until it was just right.
His favorite; our favorite,
this simple dish that came to stand for home and love and warmth.
Now as months go by I wonder
will I ever make it again? I must. There are grandchildren.
Lord, carry me over this fearsome gorge.
Will you tell him that you did?
That you brought me through?
That I cried as I mixed and stirred
and smiled when it was done.

Memory Loss

A good friend who lost her husband after a lengthy illness told me, "I forgot how to knit. I picked it up, looked at it, and put it down. I was so relieved when I found out that happens sometimes with grief; I thought something was really wrong." She went on to tell me that the skill returned a few weeks later and all was well. Just knowing kept her safe from panic and concern.

It may be well to generalize this a little. You may have other quirky things that seem concerning; Difficulty focusing, just feeling, as they say, "at loose ends." If those things happen, just relax. Your whole world just changed. A little chaos is normal.

Fatigue

So you are tired and wonder why? I expect you have been working pretty hard lately, at the very least in your head. Of course you are tired, rest. Sleep late, take bubble baths, linger over a cup of coffee, and don't worry if the house work goes begging for a few days. You have been walking on the edge of the abyss and it was hard work. We've already talked some about your diet. Perhaps here would be a good place to add a note. Unless your diet is exceptionally well balanced, buy a good multiple vitamin supplement and take it every day.

Acceptance

I wish that I could tell you that one day you will magically wake up, all will be well, and you will no longer be sad or angry or trying to change what has happened. I wish I could, but I can't.

What I can tell you is slowly you will move toward the place where sad and angry no longer defines who you are. Acceptance doesn't mean you like what happened, nor does it mean you no longer miss your mate or loved one. Nothing can change who they were or the part they played in who you have become. Somewhere, however, you will be able to remember…and smile instead of cry. You will look forward, instead of back. Slowly, the flowers in the garden again have color, and it matters what you wear: Life, again begins.

Survival Tips
- Allow tears and laughter. It is easy to work hard at not feeling. Resist.
- Remember it is a journey and sometimes there are turns and detours. Like life, grief work can sometimes be messy and unpredictable. Just accept it and go on.

- Don't set time limits on the process. Once I asked a very wise lady, "When will I ever quit crying?" She told me, "When you are done."
- Rest when you need to. Grieving can be hard work.
- Get out of the house. Fresh air and exercise can do wonders.
- Do something for someone else.

What a Friend Can Do to Help

- Don't rush or judge what your friend is going through. Everyone has a different pace.
- Don't try to figure it out. Just when you have decided it's all over and your friend is finally through, anger or tears in the middle of nowhere will erupt. It doesn't have to make sense; it just is what it is.

Points to Ponder

> *Whither shall I go from thy spirit? Or whither shall I flee from thy presence? If I ascend up into heaven, thou art there: if I make my bed in hell, behold, thou art there. If I take the wings of the morning, and dwell in the uttermost parts of the sea; Even there shall thy hand lead me, and thy right hand shall hold me.*
>
> **—Psalm 139:7–10**

This verse reminds me I am not alone. Never. He is with me now, He was with me then, and He will be with me evermore. I can face whatever comes.

Sometimes it's the little things that trip you up. This is a story from my niece who lost her husband from a heart attack at fifty. Read her story (as posted in her blog). New widows can be difficult to understand. Sometimes the things that make us cry seem trivial, even silly. But even meatloaf can be a trigger when it was your hubby's favorite dish.

How Can Meatloaf Make You Cry?

Meatloaf was one of Larry's favorite meals. I was constantly working on a way to make it better because I wasn't crazy about it, but he loved it. And if I was gone for a weekend, he almost always made meatloaf with venison. But I think he tried everything in the cabinet to make it "his" way, usually pretty spicy, or smoky, or something.

Last night, I was making Tater Tot casserole and was looking for the glass dish I always make it in. I couldn't find it anywhere! I thought maybe my wonderful cleaning girls that found my kitchen for me when Larry died had put it in a "special" place. Finally, I looked in the back of the refrigerator. There it was. And guess what was in it—meatloaf. No, it had not spoiled as it was on the top shelf and my fridge likes to "freeze" things on the top shelf.

Larry liked meatloaf; it was his favorite dish. This was a new recipe and he loved it. It was the last meal I had cooked for him. The flood gates opened, my heart ached. I just wanted him standing there complaining that we wasted the "good meatloaf" by not eating it. I may never look at that pan or meatloaf the same way.

This story speaks to me of the heartache I have known many times. Memories triggered unexpectedly by simple things. My comfort, though from many sources, is never more real than when it comes straight from the Word of God.

Chapter Eleven

Sad and Stuck

∙∙∙∙∙∙∙∙∙∙∙∙∙∙∙∙∙∙∙∙∙∙∙∙∙∙∙∙∙∙∙∙∙∙∙

I was tired, alone, and discouraged. I trusted
God for my future, but I couldn't see through the
dark surrounding me.

∙∙∙∙∙∙∙∙∙∙∙∙∙∙∙∙∙∙∙∙∙∙∙∙∙∙∙∙∙∙∙∙∙∙∙

If losses happened in predictable doses and grief stages came in neat little packages that you could open, experience, and put back on the shelf, life might never get so complicated. But it doesn't. Sometimes a second or third or fourth negative event will occur before the first can be processed. If there is too much pain, too much grief, or too few reserves, bargaining mixes with shock, anger interrupts acceptance, and everything becomes overwhelming. This chapter is about what happens when grieving gets complicated.

Grief is not an isolated event that happens to us only occasionally. Daily we experience shock, disappointment, loss, and resolution. Most events are mild and we process them without even thinking about them. We share news we think exciting and don't get the response we hoped from a friend. The new hairstyle we thought would make us look younger is a flop. The movie we couldn't wait to see is not what we expected.

Over and over our lives are pummeled with such events. Accompanied by its cellmate, disbelief, it takes a toll. We call it stress. Stress causes many reactions in the body, few of them good. At the cellular level, our bodies don't know the difference between the stress of receiving bad news and the stress of the pain from hitting our thumb with a hammer. Energy is expended and our immune system is attacked.

Two weeks after my husband's death, I found the lump that began my own battle with cancer. In the years since, I have become aware of how commonly that occurs. Caring for someone who is chronically or terminally ill is stressful even when you are totally willing and committed to the process.

I had barely completed cancer treatment when one good friend moved away and another was also diagnosed with breast cancer. My sons and daughters-in-law were also under additional stress because in addition to losing their father to cancer and my own diagnosis, each couple had an additional parent with cancer. I worried about the load they carried. I lost my job, something I never in my wildest dreams thought could happen to me. Conflict in people around me confused the issue and I was powerless to fix it.

Three years after that fateful morning when we left our drive at six AM for my husband's first colonoscopy, I was tired, alone, and discouraged. I trusted God for my future, but I couldn't see through the dark surrounding me.

One grief had piled upon another and none seemed fixable. I felt useless, defeated, and old. I wanted desperately to go home with Jesus— and my husband. Once again it wasn't God's plan.

I didn't want to feel the way I did, but I couldn't seem to change. Others didn't want me to feel that way either. I was difficult to be with, I was alternately angry, tearful, and withdrawn. Moments of feeling good were short lived.

I was fortunate to find someone who helped me work my way out of the tangle. It wasn't quick and it wasn't painless, but slowly the sun shone again and hope again returned.

Grieving may also become complicated because of multiple losses. I live less than an hour from where the EF5 tornado of 2011 ripped through the town of Joplin, Missouri. More than 150 people lost their lives and a thousand plus more were injured. Many people lost multiple loved ones, homes, and businesses. In many cases, the necessity of survival postponed dealing with loss. In the months that followed, I was in several offices where people were continuing to work because services needed to be available, yet they themselves were homeless, living with a friend, a relative, or in temporary housing.

I think sometimes that we feel we have failed if we are overcome by grief. Especially if we are Christians, we believe that we are above sadness, grief, and anger; we worry others will question our faith.

The truth is, God does promise to bring us through. His word is clear about that. Never, however, does He say it will be easy, effortless, or without complication. It is wise when we recognize the need to find someone to come along side.

You may be feeling, right now, like all is hopeless. I understand. Do not suffer in silence. We hate the word depression. Maybe we are just weak. Maybe we just need to trust God more. Maybe we just need to get out more, or take a yoga class, or eat better, or sleep less, or forget the past, or whatever. Many times depression is rooted in beliefs and behaviors that aren't good for us. That's true. However, depression happens when the serotonin levels in our brain become depleted. That's what cocaine does. Cocaine causes you to use mega amounts of serotonin all at once. That is why it feels so good. Cocaine addicts come off of cocaine in a huge depressed state, because their serotonin is all gone. Stress over long periods of time does exactly the same thing. If you have been under stress, either physical or emotional or mental, you are at risk. Sometimes medication can help get that straightened out. It may be a physical problem that needs a physical cure. Do you need to do the other things too? Absolutely. Find someone to talk to—your pastor, a grief counselor or group—someone who will help you talk about and process all of the many things that have happened. Improve your diet, rest, exercise, get out of the house, and have some fun. It's all important, and YOU are worth it.

You may be concerned that your friend or family member is not doing as well as they should with the grief process. Perhaps you can help. Listening can be an important help. Encourage them to talk about the losses. It's okay if they cry. They may need to. However, sometimes more is needed and suggesting that they see their doctor can help. It is funny but true that if we cut our arm we know to go to the doctor, but if we feel bad, somehow, we just need someone else's permission to seek help. Some of the things to look for that would signal a need for help would be:

1. Loss of interest in previous activities. Are you or your loved one isolating at home, unable or uninterested in attending church, clubs, or outings with friends? Do you think of going out but then change your mind because getting ready is just too much trouble?
2. Loss of interest in personal health or cleanliness. Is make-up a thing of the past?
3. Crying without warning or without even understanding why.
4. Thinking of or talking about dying.
5. Eating more or less than previously.
6. Sleeping excessively or seemingly not at all.
7. Confusion, memory loss, and difficulty concentrating on things, even hallucinations.
8. Multiple losses in the past year.
9. Frequent feelings or expressions of feeling guilt, anger, or anxiety.

Survival Tips

What should you do when the grief is more than you can bear? Do you wish you could feel differently but have no idea how to go about it?

Complicated grief is not failure. It is not because you are weak, crazy, or bad. It is a real condition, caused by real losses that have bombarded you faster than you have been able to repel or deal with them. It is strength, not weakness to seek help.

- Tell a trusted friend. Choose wisely however. If this is a friend who has been judgmental about your feelings in the past, they may not be the best choice. Find someone who has had previous experience with grief or knowledge of helpful resources.
- Confide in your pastor. If he is unable to help you, he may be able to help find someone who can.
- Find a grief group to attend. Check with your hospital, local hospices, cancer center, and churches. If you live in a larger city, you may have several to choose from.
- Call your local health or mental health center for referral to a counselor or group that deals with grief issues.

What a Friend Can Do to Help

- Be patient but be firm. It may be necessary for you to suggest, guide, or even take your loved one to someone who can help. They may resist. Your calm assurance that they are not bad, weak, or wrong can help.
- Do not gossip. The prayer chain does not need to know all the details. Tell them exactly what you would want said if it were you that was grieving. "Mary is grieving and needs our prayers" is quite enough.
- If you must seek guidance about what to do to help, be selective. Go to your pastor, talk with a friend who is skilled or has experience and who can be trusted.
- Take care that you are not overheard by children or others in your home who may not understand or who may not be able to keep confidences.

Points to Ponder

I waited patiently for the LORD; and he inclined unto me, and heard my cry.

He brought me up also out of an horrible pit, out of the miry clay, and set my feet upon a rock, and established my goings.

And he hath put a new song in my mouth, even praise unto our God: many shall see it, and fear, and shall trust in the LORD.

—Psalm 40:1–3

I wish that I could say I always waited patiently for the Lord. I didn't. There have been many days when I have been very impatient for a new song; longed to feel the solid rock beneath my feet. Depression is a hard place to be. It is an even harder place to stay. Sometimes, as painful as it is, it is also an easy place to return.

This verse is a reminder of God's promise to bring us up out of the pit of despair. The solid rock is Jesus. Sometimes we must cling to Him so tightly we have no ability to do anything else. Those days are not foreign to me.

I remember one particularly bad season when it just seemed as if I could not rise above the mire pulling me down. Everywhere I turned, happy people laughed, couples held hands, those in the other pews at church appeared to have victory, and I only had tears.

I remember once, many years ago, going through a difficult season. I had asked a dear friend, "When will I ever quit crying?" Her response was "When you are done."

Looking back, I know that both times, God allowed me to cry until I was done, all the while guarding and protecting so that I did not slip to an unreachable depth in that awful clay. Then, when I was done, He lifted me, and the new song came. It will come for you too, trust Him. Know that it is okay to feel what you feel, cry when you need to cry, all the while knowing that you are never out of reach of the master's hand.

Chapter Twelve

Children and Grandchildren

· ·

Where Did Grandpa Go?

Such an innocent question, but its speaking causes my heart to wretch within me.

GONE! I think GONE!

Tears form like stinging nettles in my eyes.

But she is looking at me with the look I have seen so many times in this past few months.

At three, the explanation is hard. What will she understand? How can she comprehend?

I open my mouth to speak, the words don't come.

And then I hear.

"Heaven Grandma. Grandpa went to heaven … with Jesus!"

She is excited to tell me the answer she now remembers as she runs to my lap.

"See my new dolly," she says, content now to return to the here and now!

My heart sees him smile.

"That's my granddaughter," he says to Jesus.

"I know," he hears in response.

"Your new dolly is perfectly beautiful," I say.

· ·

I have been blessed with very precious grandchildren. Each of them tied in special ways to our journey through cancer's dark doors.

Blake was seven when his grandpa died. He carries the memories for them all. He is sensitive and kind, speaking on occasion of "missing grandpa." Not long after the funeral, he and I sat at our local diner for our traditional pancake breakfast after he spent the night. We talked about grandpa, and he reached out his little hand to me, put it carefully on my shoulder, and said, "It's okay Grandma, I will be here for you." Tears filled my eyes then, as they do now as I write.

Anna was only three. The day that she was born was the first day we saw the surgeon. We drove from the appointment to the hospital. What a bittersweet day that was. We had just scheduled the procedure that would lead us down a yet unknown road, and she was our first very precious granddaughter.

Olivia, three months younger, was also three. She is the little girl with the *Where did Grandpa Go* question in the poem above. Today Anna and Olivia have fleeting memories. Memories I try to keep alive with pictures and stories. I know they will fade soon and it makes me sad.

Lily was only eighteen months and she has no memories even now. She is a bright and happy little girl who always has a story to tell. She, like all the others, would be her grandpa's joy if he were here. Josie, born three months after his death, while I was already in the throes of my own cancer treatment, was my signal to go on. He never saw her, though he knew she was on the way. She is my name sake, Josie Fae. Each birthday that we celebrate takes me back to the night I went alone to the hospital to first hold her in my arms.

Death and illness are hard on so many levels. One of those is the children. Death is sad and sometimes hard to understand. Hard, when you are a grown-up, confusing and possibly frightening when you are a child. Understanding how a child views death at different ages and stages may help you know how to explain and deal with it with the children in your life. I said help, because each child is unique, each with their own personalities, thoughts, fears, and feelings.

When preparing to write this chapter on the effects of death and grieving in children and young adults, I began researching the topic. In doing so I came across a website sponsored by the Vita Innovative Hospice Care and articles written by Robin Fiorelli, VITAS Director of Bereavement and Volunteers. In reading her work, I was able to see the experiences I had observed in our own children being supported in her work. In most cases herein, the examples are my own; however ideas from her work were used to further explain the processes and concepts behind the behaviors. I would highly recommend this site for further reading on this subject. Specifically, the article "Children's Developmental Stages: Concepts of Death and Responses to Grief" was most helpful. (See http://www.vitas.com/Services/ LearnAboutHospice/BereavementSupport/   GriefandBereavement/ ChildrensDevelopmentalStagesConceptsofDeath.aspx.)

Infant to Age Two

Babies think only in the present. What is seen is real, what is not seen is possibly forgotten. They do not have the ability to think abstractly. Death will not be a concept understood. What they will be affected by is the change in the environment, the difference in who is holding or rocking them to sleep. They may sense the sadness and grief in others and react to it, even though they do not know what it is.

Their reactions may include anxiety, crying, irritability, and change in sleep patterns, eating habits, and activity levels.

Preschool (Age Two to Four)

This age is still unable to understand abstract concepts like death or forever. Death is seen as something that is reversible. Though they are beginning to remember things that are not in view (Can I have a cookie from the jar?), they are unable to completely understand the concept of gone forever. They may continue to look for the person and ask when they are coming home. They may want to know how the deceased can eat or breathe.

In the last stages of his illness, my husband had developed a craving for chocolate. A fondness he shared with the grandkids. When they came to see him, he always gave them candy. It became such a big deal that when he died, we added a few chocolate bars to his casket. On one occasion not long after my husband's funeral, one of the three-year-old granddaughters remembered that and her conversation with me was a perfect example of how she saw death.

Olivia: "Grandpa died."

Me: "Yes, he did."

Olivia: "Grandma, do you remember that big box they put him in?"

Me: "Yes, I do."

Olivia "Grandma, do you remember that we put some candy bars in there?"

Me: "Yes, Olivia, we did do that."

Olivia: "Well, do you think he has eaten those all by now?"

Grief reactions at this age may be brief but very intense. Unable to completely comprehend what has happened yet sensing the sadness of others, they may act out with crying, whining, tantrums, or withdrawal. It is a time to hold, comfort, give a little slack, and even offer distractions. Be prepared to offer short, intense reassurance one minute and watch giggling and somersaults in the next. Often, by the time you have gathered your wits to try and explain, the moment has changed and the "present" with its distraction of a favorite toy has taken over.

Early Childhood (Age Four to Seven)

This can be a difficult age for a child dealing with the death of a loved one. Still unable to think abstractly, death is often seen as temporary and reversible. They may connect things that are not connected, especially if things are not explained to them. They may also believe that they are responsible. "It's all my fault, I was mad at grandpa." Children this age are pretty self-centered. The world revolves around them and what they are doing. They believe that they can control it; that what they think happens. They may believe that it is possible to avoid death if you do the right things.

It is not uncommon for them to look for the deceased, or ask where they are, or when they will return. Questions regarding the person or the death may continue to be voiced. At just barely five, our granddaughter heard us talking about the funeral visitation she had attended with us the day before. "You mean that room where he was dead?" It was clear from her expression that she did not expect that he was going to remain "dead," but that it was a temporary situation.

It may be difficult to know how a child of this age is feeling as they may not express their feelings very readily. They may even appear not to be affected at all. Often they take cues from the adults around them as to how to act. If the adults are doing a very "good job" of holding in their feelings so as not to upset the child, they may, in fact, be hindering the child's ability to feel the loss and grieve properly.

How a child reacts to death may also be in part due to their own personality. Even at a very young age, children exhibit their own unique beliefs and ways of dealing with issues. Recently we attended a family member's funeral. Now at the ages of eight and six, my granddaughters reacted very differently. The older, when given the choice, declined "viewing" the body and casket. It seemed not to matter at all to her. It was as if, even at her young age of eight, she understood that he was not there within the physical shell. Her sister, just a bit younger, is the curious sort. She wanted to see and she had many questions. She wanted to know all and understand all. I was pleased that the parents dealt with each child individually, allowing the distancing and answering the questions. More than anything, children need adults who will treat them as real people and deal with their questions and feelings with honesty and respect.

Expressing their grief through play is common. Funerals and themes of loss or death may be noted in their play and playacting. While it may be upsetting to the adult, it is in fact helpful to the child.

I have a grandson who has Asperger's Syndrome. He was very close to his grandpa. He wrote the following. I believe it is helpful in understanding what children are aware of and remember about the death experience. Notice how Blake relates his grandfather's Air Force experience to his need to control his own emotions. Blake also hits on an important fact to remember. Kids know, kids feel, kids need to talk about what they know and feel. If you can't, find someone who can.

"Hi I'm Blake. I am twelve years old and I have Asperger's. I was seven when I lost my Grandpa Orin. I had no idea what was going on. When I went to his house he wasn't there. Even his bed was gone. I didn't understand. I asked 'Where's grandpa.' It seemed like no one answered my question. I guess they didn't know what to say to me."

"When I did see grandpa, he was in what I called back then a big wood body holder. Now I know it is called a casket. I felt upset but he was in the Air Force so I didn't cry. It was hard for me to hold back the tears though and right when we left the church I cried cause I had lost some one that I loved dearly and after the funeral I decided to help grandma with her work. So it's not easy with a special need kids. It's not easy for any kids. I thought if you knew what it was like for me; it would help you help your kids. Let them know what is going on and if they want to talk about it let them. You can also have them go to a counselor to help them."

Eight to Ten

In this age range, a child begins to see death as more permanent and final. They still may want to see it as reversible. Many questions may surface. Curiosity about death, the funeral procedure, cremation, and burial are common. Unaware as yet of the "social etiquette," their questions may seem forward, direct, and candid.

Death is something that is seen as happening to old people. Death may be seen as avoidable with the right efforts or as punishment. Confusion and inability to completely comprehend the concept of death can result in anxiety.

Children in this age range may appear to have little concern about the death, they may simply withdraw and hide their feelings, or they may act out their anger and sadness in misbehavior. It is not uncommon for children this age to worry or fear others may die. Be aware that anger and sadness may cause difficulty concentrating in school. If you see signs of depression such as changes in eating, sleeping patterns, loss of interest in activities, or withdrawal, it would be good to find someone who can help the child talk about the grief they are experiencing. Regression to an earlier developmental stage could occur. Oppositional behavior may be common. Something isn't right, they just don't quite know what or why or how to fix it. Death may be playacted especially in children who have difficulty expressing feelings verbally. This is not a bad thing and should not be discouraged as it is often the way that children work through the experience. Children may also assume tasks performed by the deceased, or adopt mannerisms of the deceased. This is a way to maintain some contact with the person they have lost.

Regressing into earlier behavior patterns may be a way for the child to elicit the nurturing that is needed. Fear that other significant adults in their life may leave them is not uncommon. As with the preschooler, tolerance, cuddling, and reassurance along with honest answers to their questions is helpful in helping the child move through the grief.

Pre-Adolescent (Age Ten to Twelve)

My personal experience with older children experiencing death is limited. According to Theresa Huntley in her book, *Helping Children Grieve*, pre-adolescents conceive of death in much the same way as children in the middle years with a few additions. "Pre-adolescents are in the process of establishing their own identity, increasing their independence from their parents and other adults, and increasing their dependence on their peer group. In understanding death, pre-adolescents attempt to understand both the biological and emotional process of death. They are, however, more able to understand the facts surrounding the death of someone than they are the feelings surrounding the death" (Huntley 1991, 17).

Survival Tips

- Find comfort in your children and grandchildren. Stop what you are doing, or thinking, and just watch them. In the innocence of their play and the mysteries of the many thoughts that spill from their lips as they discover, learn, and participate in the world around them, they will show you how to love and move forward. Don't miss it. Don't fail to learn from it. It is one of your lifelines.

- Allow and plan for the children around you. Your life may be busy, or it may have seemed to slow to a stop. Either way, chances are, you need to play. If the weather allows, take them for a walk. Together, notice the leaves, the rainbow, and the acorns on the ground. Let them talk. Listen. Hold their hand. Laugh, while they run ahead to jump a puddle or the crack in the sidewalk. Tell them that you love them; tell them sometimes you are sad. Allow them to be. And if it works, get an ice-cream cone on the way home.

What a Friend Can Do to Help

- This can be a stressful time for kids. Offer to take them to the park or to your house to play. They may benefit more than you know from the sense of normality that the time away can provide.

- Be patient with them. Respond to misbehavior with "I know this has been a hard time for you and you are sad. Would you like to tell me about it?" It may be easier for them to talk if they are not afraid they will make mommy or grandma sadder if they do.

- Understand if they are silent. Affirm that you understand things have been tough and it's okay to feel angry, and then offer a distraction. "How about we go check on those baby kittens I was telling you about?"
- Offer assurances that the adults in their life will be okay. "Grandma is sad right now, but she loves you and one day soon she will be ready to play with you again."

Points to Ponder

> *"And he said unto him, My lord knoweth that the children are tender ..."*
>
> **—Genesis 33:13**

In this passage of scripture, Jacob is pleading with his brother Esau to allow his family to travel slowly because of the hardship on the small children with them. We need to plead that case for our small children as well. This is a difficult time and they are tender. Value them and protect them.

Chapter Thirteen

Practical Problems

....

FURNACE FILTERS
He always knew when it was time.
"Get the 18x22, two of them, so we
will have an extra," he would say.
Where do they go, these fiber sheets
with cardboard frames?
I never looked, never knew.
Why?
Why didn't I know about this thing
that to him was so routine?
Will I ever be okay in this world where
it takes two, while I am now alone?

....

New Tasks, Responsibilities, and Decisions
How drastic will the changes affect you? Consider a wife whose
husband has been an over-the-road truck driver. For years she has paid

the bills, called the plumber when she could not fix the faucet herself, gone to school programs, church, and the dentist alone—well, alone except for the three children. Her outside-the-home job as a social worker at the local hospital has introduced her to the inner workings of the medical field, the local, state, and national resources, problem solving, and the available local support systems.

In contrast, the wife who raised three children, with a loving and supportive husband who handled all the financial and practical issues, made attending school and church functions a priority, and often took the kids to their appointments because "mom needed to stay home with the other two."

Please do not assume that I am saying that one situation is better or preferable to the other. I am not. Differences in our life experiences, however, will affect how we may be prepared to deal with widowhood.

A second factor is our basic personalities. If you are familiar with personality typing, you are likely already having scenarios going off in your head. If not, here is a brief explanation.

Usually personality types are divided into four groups. The first two are made up of the leaders and the people persons. Leaders see the vision, the big picture, but aren't so good at the detail. They may or may not be socially inclined. People Persons love to be with others and are particularly good at implementing the visions and motivating others.

Steady, detail-oriented workers make up the last two types. They work very well when they know what to do, how to do it, and have clear instructions.

Left alone to manage it all, the first groups will soon have figured out where their life needs to go from here and will appear to have it all together. It is quite likely, however, that they forget to pay the electric bill, don't notice the leaky faucet, and except in a crisis … i.e., the electricity just got turned off … they wonder why you are so concerned with all those details. By contrast, the persons who are detail oriented may not be good at making life changing decisions, or even getting out of the house.

A third factor is how quickly the person became responsible for the total picture. My husband was two years into his illness before he lost the ability to do most of the things he had previously done, so I was able to slowly learn and absorb his previous tasks. My niece, whose husband died suddenly at fifty, became immediately responsible for all of it, including their farm and animals.

Whatever your situation, or that of your friends, there are some basic things that you will need to address.

Finances

I have previously mentioned that at the very least, it is likely your income will be cut in half. This must be dealt with pretty quickly. Having good life insurance coverage can make a huge difference as to how you will manage. Even if you have already been handling these resources, I would encourage you to seek the advice and assistance of someone who is skilled in this area. It may be a trusted family member or friend. It may be someone you hire. I know from experience that grief can lead to unwise decisions. Having someone who at the very least can just be a good ear is invaluable.

Legal Issues

Some things in today's modern computer age will happen for you. The funeral director will order the death certificates. You will need to tell them how many you need. You should plan to have one for each life insurance policy. I ordered three extra and have used two of them.

The Social Security Administration will know almost immediately of a death. I believe this is also a function of your funeral director.

Wills, IRAs, bank accounts, car and other personal property titles, deeds, land titles, utilities, phone, cable, and Internet accounts are all things that will need to be changed. It is also good to consider whether you should include someone, such as one of your children, on these accounts and titles.

Housing Issues

If you can, you should stay where you are for at least a year. That's the standard advice and I think it is good. I didn't, and I regretted it later. What now seems unbearable—the memories, where he sat, where she cooked—will later turn into comforts and its good if you can hang around for that.

Relationships

This is a tough one. I think the "wait a year" is good advice, but I have seen many who seem to be in good relationships much sooner. I am not sure there is a "time" that is right for everyone. If you are a Christian, talk to the Lord about it. Let Him guide you. I believe it was better for me to learn to lean completely on Him before I even considered one else.

At this stage in my life, I am content to be alone. It has a lot of downsides, but it also has advantages. As I write, I am sitting in my den with the fireplace going. I got up at five-thirty … and no I don't always do that … I have been writing since, with a few breaks to eat, read my Bible, watch the snow storm outside, and fold some laundry. I woke no one in the process, cooked for no one, and am quite comfy still in my pajamas. Lunch will be whatever, and whenever I decide, and no, I haven't made the bed or washed the dishes.

This hasn't always been the way I felt, and it may not be the way I feel next week. Perhaps my experience will help you.

Shortly after my husband's death I yearned to meet someone. I even checked out the online "meet people" sites. Fearing I would disgrace my husband's memory, I didn't pursue that, and within a few weeks realized I didn't want or need another mate; I wanted and needed the one I lost.

About three years into widowhood, I again thought a new mate would be a good idea. Over time, I met a couple of people, considered it, but then again became okay with my single status. That's where I am today, but it could change. God may choose to put someone in my life this very day, and if He does, well, who knows.

All that said, go slow. You can never replace what you had. If you do build a new life with someone else, it could be better. It might be worse. It will, however, never be the same. Allow yourself the time to accept that before you move on.

Developing a New Support System

Single people and married people may not mix
This was a sad realization for me. I wanted to continue spending time with my married friends, but it just didn't work. I am not totally sure why, but the best advice I have is accept it and go on.

Some people will not be comfortable with your grief
They just won't. It isn't right or wrong, it just is. Again, accept it and go on. Your friendship with them might pick back up later, and if it does, don't hold a grudge because they weren't there for you. They just weren't, and it was because they couldn't, not because they didn't want to.

Your freedom to pursue new interests will cause you to develop new friends
Because I have the freedom to schedule and do things without concern about leaving my husband at home or not cooking a meal, I have been able to do things that I would have otherwise not done. One of those was joining the writers group that was instrumental in my writing this book.

Old hobbies and interests can be rejuvenated
An exciting thing for me has been the time I have had to restart doing things I had previously enjoyed and put aside because of time constraints. Sewing was one such hobby. Having learned young, I used the skill all through my life, even sewing many of our clothing. The craft had lain idle for many years, however, as work and illness took my time.

Now I often spend many hours in my bedroom-turned-sewing studio, creating ruffled skirts, doll clothes, funky hats, and more.

Think about what you used to love and do it again. I have found comfort in regressing to old activities and implementing them in new and fun ways. I bet you will too!

Survival Tips

- Try something new.
- Go somewhere you've never been before.
- Tell your grandkids lots of stories.
- Talk to someone you trust before making life changing decisions.

What a Friend Can Do to Help

- Read this whole chapter. Be sensitive to the personality and needs of your friend or family member. I don't know if I would have made different decisions if someone had really voiced their concern, but I hope I might have.
- How to be there for a friend when your natural instinct is to withdraw: It is hard to be with someone who is hurting without trying to fix the situation. We want to do something to stop the pain. We want to help. Often the one thing that we can do to help is the one thing that we are afraid we will do if we stay there. Sound crazy? Well it isn't.

When you are with someone who is hurting, we often fear we will not know what to say. We fear we will just sit there and say nothing. Interestingly, that is often best. Oh, you might say, "I don't know what to say, but I'm here," or "I don't know what to say, but I am here to listen." You could say, "Tell me about how you are feeling right now," or "tell me about him" or "what is your biggest worry." Ask questions that aren't answered by yes or no and just let the person talk. They will find their own answers, if they even need one.

Points to Ponder

> *Bear you one another's burdens, and so fulfill the law of Christ.*
>
> **—Galatians 6:2**

> *A new commandment I give unto you, that ye love one another; as I have loved you, that ye also love one another.*
>
> **—John 13:34**

In Galatians we are told to bear one another's burdens and to do it in a way that fulfills the law of Christ. In the Old Testament the law was written, detailed, strict, and unforgiving in its interpretation. Christ gave a new directive. In John 13:34, Jesus tells us the law is new. He tells us we are to love as He loves. Gone are the days when following the letter of the law, with or without a good attitude, would suffice. Loving, as Jesus did, meant real concern, real activity. He didn't just say, "Wow, I am sorry you are sick." He healed. He didn't say, "Sorry you didn't catch any fish today." He said, "Cast your net on the other side," and it was filled. And ultimately, He didn't just say "Well, guys, time for me to go home, see you later if you can figure out how to get there." No, instead He said, "In my Father's house are many mansions: if it were not so, I would have told you. I go to prepare a place for you. And if I go and prepare a place for you, I will come again, and receive you unto myself; that where I am, there ye may be also" (John 14:2–3).

It is hard to be alone, yet it can be an opportunity, one each of us can use to grow in Christ and in our service to each other. It is not easy to put someone else's needs above our own, yet it is what Christ meant when He said we were to love each other as we loved ourselves.

What can you do today to help someone in need? Have you even stopped to consider what that might be? Maybe, God wants you to turn off the TV and pray. Maybe He wants you to go mow a yard. Do it.

Is it an easy thing? No. It is easier to turn the TV louder so you don't have to hear the other message. It is easier to say, "later" or "oh, well" and ignore the need.

Am I thinking of only friends and family here? No, not at all; one of the best things you can do, now that you are alone and the responsibilities of caregiving have been lifted, is to begin to reach out and love others as Christ has commanded. As, in the past months, others have reached out in love to you.

Chapter Fourteen

Old Memories
and New Traditions

· ·

HIS TIES

Like steady soldiers they stand.
Straight and quiet just inside the closet door
Each with its special memory to tell
His favorite and mine,
The one he wore the night our son was married.
I look at them tenderly and remember.
Sweet memories of yesterday
flood my mind and heart.
Tears. Will they ever stop?
And then you remind me
Lord that he is with you.
Tomorrow is not so far. I can see it just ahead.
Thank You Lord,
For giving me the courage to remember

The good things that these ties represent;
For the tears which cleanse,
But oh Lord most of all
For your sweet promise of a day to come.
••••••••••••••••••••••••••••••••

Remembering

The further I am from the moment of loss, the more desperately I want to remember. Memories, that at first were painful, have now become precious. I wish that I could have captured every word, every look, and every experience; the good ones, the bad ones, the boring, and exciting ones. Sometimes they are there, in a photograph, a valentine card, a memento, but sometimes they are not. My son inherited his grandpa's tractor—the one that he remembers seeing delivered to their farm many years ago. A few years ago, in a freak accident, the tractor was burned. Lovingly, Mike restored it, photographing it in all its various stages. Then he asked if we had any photograph of grandpa on that tractor. We didn't. Many years ago cameras weren't used as frequently as they are today. They recorded special events like birthdays and graduations, not field work and farm equipment. It has made me very aware, now, of how I record our family history. I look more often for the unrecorded things that will later be the memories my children will cherish.

What Do I Keep and What Goes Out the Door?

It is a very personal decision when it comes to dealing with the personal belongings of your loved one. I do think that it is important you do most of the sorting and decision making if at all possible. I have found priceless mementos mixed in with all the rest. Priceless, that is, to me, because it triggered a long forgotten pleasant memory. Some things will hold little value for you; others will stir your heart. I found it easy to empty the closet of shirts and pants and underwear. His ties will stay with me always. My husband for many years owned and operated his own photography studio. His ties stirred my remembrances of that time of our lives. I don't want to give them up. I think perhaps I will make a quilt. A particular shirt had significance to his sister and she took it home to treasure.

One possible solution to all the items and mementos which hold meaning but are too numerous to keep is to make a photo album of them. Photograph them and put them in an album with a description beside each one as to its meaning. It is so easy and inexpensive now to select and print a quality book online that it is a great solution. Picmonkey.com and Shutterfly.com are two sources online, but many now offer these for reasonable prices.

Photographs

Photographs are still a huge issue at my house. I have hundreds, enough that they fill several albums and an old trunk. He was a photographer. I find that some of the commercial shots, while of nothing I care about, hold special meaning because of the memories of his working with those customers. Maybe I should just do a little book of his work, hmm?

Whatever you do with them, photographs can be great memory joggers. Now when I am feeling nostalgic and want to relive some of our old times, the photograph trunk and a pot of coffee make for a cozy afternoon.

Recently, my son Mike and I have embarked on a new venture. It all started with the photo book Mike made of our recent vacation and talk of coming plans for my mother's ninety-fifth birthday celebration. He said, "Mom, you write her story, and I will do the pictures. We can make a book of her life." So, using e-mail to query all the kids, grandkids, and great grandkids, I have gathered memories and am writing them into the story. Soon we will have it ready to go and I will begin on another, perhaps their dad's this time.

Sharing His Things

Many people have known your loved one and may have memories that are different than you. One thing that you might say to them before your elimination process is this: "I know that you loved _____ too. I am going through things to decide what to keep. I would like you to have something of his. What things might I find that have a special meaning to you?" They may not have any particular thing, but you may also be surprised to find that something you thought worthless indeed held special memories.

Feelings

Anger, sadness, tears. Why are they all here again? Do not be surprised when this process triggers a few tears. It should. Some of these tears should be happy tears, however, as you enjoy the memories of special times together. One set of items, now stored safely in my memory box, are the name badges he wore at various times in his life.

His US Air Force pin, the ID badge from the University, the name badge from our Square Dance club where together we were presidents—all these can take me on a trip back through time.

Telling Stories—Children Love to Listen

Few things can make me smile like a grandchild saying, "Tell us about the time that grandpa ____." They are still young now, and stories can be simple and short, or long and elaborate. They don't care. They giggle at the telling and want them over and over.

So you don't think you could do that? Not a storyteller? Try anyway. Sit down with your daughter, son, grandchild, niece, or nephew on your lap (make snuggling a specialty) and just remember. "Did I ever tell you about the time grandpa and I went camping?" "Do you know what your mom liked best about Saturday mornings?" "Your uncle was my brother and when we were little we used to. . ."

I tell them frequently, "Grandpa would have loved you so much if he were here. He used to hold you on his lap and you would play." Blake, our oldest grandchild, remembers his grandpa. Rarely does he visit that we do not talk about him.

Anna and the Ribbons is one of our favorite stories. It had its origin after the cancer and the medications had made it impossible for us to go out to eat. Mike and Emily, our son and daughter-in-law had gone to eat at a favorite barbeque. Ribs were one of my husband's favorite foods, and Anna, just two and barely talking, was so excited when she got back. In she came, bag in hand, declaring that she had brought ribbons for grandpa to eat. What fun they had that night, and what a precious memory. We remind Anna of this night whenever we happen to be eating ribs. They are, incidentally, still one of Anna's favorite foods. It is good for them to remember and reminisce; it's even better for me that someone remembers him and says so.

Writing your Story

If you are in the habit of keeping a journal, it will be easy to begin including your thoughts and memories in it. If not, it may take some discipline to begin. There are several ways to record your thoughts and memories and I will suggest a few, but the important thing is just to start. One thing that has happened for me is the urgency to write down the things about him and our lives that I want our kids to know. Our history, clues to his personality, thoughts, and dreams. Where they came from and where we hoped they would go. Writing can accomplish that in a way that preserves those things that are dear to you, and holds them, until your children and grandchildren are ready to hear them.

Write His

We did a photo story for my husband's funeral. If it is done in a program like Microsoft® PowerPoint, it is easy to go back and add information, stories, etc. It's hard to do that in the normal three days before a funeral, and it's really not for the masses, but for you and for his family. The story will provide a wonderful record and memory of his life and be a healing project for you.

Tell God

Perhaps your journal just needs to be for you and God. That's okay, He wants to hear.

Survival Tips

- Share items with your kids, grandkids, and other relatives that will mean something to them.
- Take a picture of the many things that remind you of him and make a photo book. Add a story so it's there forever.
- Do things when you are ready. Don't force yourself.

What a Friend Can Do to Help?

- Listen.
- When you think of the one who is gone, say so.

Points to Ponder

> *And God shall wipe away all tears from their eyes; and there shall be no more death, neither sorrow, nor crying, neither shall there be any more pain: for the former things are passed away.*
>
> **—Revelations 21:4**

One day we will stand on that golden street, walk beside the crystal sea, and hear the wind in lush green trees. Our hearts will be full of joy and peace, and the sorrows of this world will be a distant memory. I long for that day. Still, I am here, and this day I choose to have joy where I am. I can enjoy again the giggles of the little girls in my life and know their tender touch as they crawl into my lap for one last hug before going home. I can wait for spring once more and marvel when tender crocus peek their heads from winter soil. Today, I will seek to be a better servant, a kinder person, a more joyful friend.

Moving Forward

• •

Eat Ice Cream for Supper
I have no need to rush right home today.
No one is there. Sometimes this is difficult.
Today I find it freeing.
I wander around the local flea market
looking for a forgotten treasure.
I eat ice cream for supper.
Finally, weary of the day, I enter
the door where no one greets.
I don't hang up my coat and I don't do dishes.
The book I left last night lay
beckoning on the table.
I respond.
Guilt touches me but only for an instant.
Today it is just me and that's okay.

• •

Purpose Where None Seems to Exist

My world has changed some in the six years since my husband's home-going. And there are days that I miss him terribly. But mostly my life is rich and full. I am "Nothergrandma" to Anna, Lily, and Josie, and just plain Grandma to Blake and Olivia, Logan, Lucas, and Lily Ann. I am filled with purpose as I am allowed to participate in their dreams. Lily Ann is a gymnast, Anna a dancer. Lily Claire is learning to play the piano. Blake is our artist and Olivia our sweetheart; Lucas never fails to bring me a hug and Josie a smile. Logan is our quiet one, ever vigilant.

I lead a Bible study now, and am blessed to be able to share God's Holy Word and prayer with the dear ladies who attend.

Sewing, learned many years ago, in that same 4-H club where I met my sweetheart, has provided hours of pleasure and helpful income. I make ruffled skirts for little girls, and my heart sings when, as on a recent occasion, one of my granddaughters came running out of my sewing room saying, "Grandma, Grandma, there is a skirt in there that I just love, and I think it is my size!" And I write. In the depths of my sorrow, months after my loss, God gave me the poems that are woven through the pages of this book. Tucked quietly in my heart and on the chip in my computer they waited patiently to be used.

I hadn't planned to be a writer. Never thought I would write a book. I tagged along with my cousin to that Christian Writer's Fellowship meeting down at the public library. Mostly I hung around and enjoyed the fellowship part. God had other plans.

I look back now on all that has happened and I understand that we are all a beautiful symphony, orchestrated by a wondrous God. I have loved Him for many years. I have trusted Him with all I have. He alone knew that without the pain this book could not come forth. I hope in reading it, it will bless you as in the writing I have been blessed.

What can you do when you are where I was? Where I am?

Our situations may not be identical, but the process is:

- Do the grief work
- Explore your options

- Ask and wait
- Find a new normal

Cry if you want to. Laugh when you can.
And when it feels right—***eat ice cream for supper***.

What the Bible Says

It often seems to me that if someone wanted to know for sure that they were going to heaven when they died, that they would care more about what the Bible says than about anything I could say. God's Word is in italics. All scriptures are from the King James Version.

Heaven and earth and all things on it came from God

> *In the beginning God created the heaven and the earth.*
> **—Genesis 1:1**

> *In the beginning was the Word, and the Word was with God, and the Word was God. The same was in the beginning with God All things were made by him; and without him was not anything made that was made.*
> **—John 1:1–3**

Including man, woman, and marriage

> *And the LORD God formed man of the dust of the ground,*
> *and breathed into his nostrils the breath of life; and man*
> *became a living soul.*
>
> *And the LORD God said, It is not good that the man*
> *should be alone; I will make him an help meet for him.*
>
> —Genesis 2:7, 18

> *And the LORD God caused a deep sleep to fall upon Adam,*
> *and he slept: and he took one of his ribs, and closed up the*
> *flesh instead thereof; And the rib, which the LORD God*
> *had taken from man, made he a woman, and brought her*
> *unto the man.*
>
> —Genesis 2:21–22

> *And they were both naked, the man and his wife, and*
> *were not ashamed.*
>
> —Genesis 2:25

They lived in paradise until they sinned

> *Now the serpent was more subtil than any beast of the field*
> *which the LORD God had made. And he said unto the*
> *woman, Yea, hath God said, Ye shall not eat of every tree*
> *of the garden? And the woman said unto the serpent, We*
> *may eat of the fruit of the trees of the garden: But of the*
> *fruit of the tree which is in the midst of the garden, God*
> *hath said, Ye shall not eat of it, neither shall ye touch it,*
> *lest ye die. And the serpent said unto the woman, Ye shall*
> *not surely die: For God doth know that in the day ye eat*
> *thereof, then your eyes shall be opened, and ye shall be as*
> *gods, knowing good and evil. And when the woman saw*

that the tree was good for food, and that it was pleasant to the eyes, and a tree to be desired to make one wise, she took of the fruit thereof, and did eat, and gave also unto her husband with her; and he did eat. And the eyes of them both were opened, and they knew that they were naked; and they sewed fig leaves together, and made themselves aprons.

—Genesis 3:1–7

Sin required that blood be shed

Unto Adam also and to his wife did the LORD God make coats of skins, and clothed them.

—Genesis 3:21

Two thousand years

For two thousand years, God's chosen people, Israel, were required to sacrifice a perfect animal every year to pay for their sins. This was according to the law given to them by God through Moses and the prophets. That law is recorded in Deuteronomy and Leviticus.

Finally God's plan for the salvation of man was fulfilled. One night about two thousand years ago, a baby was born in a stable in Bethlehem to a virgin named Mary, fulfilling all prophesies about the coming Messiah. That story is in Luke chapter two.

For unto you is born this day in the city of David a Saviour, which is Christ the Lord.

—Luke 2:11

Thirty-three years later, on a cross on Calvary, Jesus Christ was crucified for crimes he did not commit. He did so because the plan was that his blood shed on that cross would pay the sin debt for all people before and after him who believed in him and accepted his gift of salvation.

*But he was wounded for our transgressions; he was bruised
for our iniquities: the chastisement of our peace was upon
him; and with his stripes we are healed.*

—Isaiah 53:5

Our spiritual condition is explained in these verses in Romans

As it is written, There is none righteous, no, not one:

—Romans 3:10

All have sinned and come short of the glory of God;

—Romans 3:23

Jesus, God's only begotten son, was willing to pay the price for us

*For he hath made him to be sin for us, who knew no sin;
that we might be made the righteousness of God in Him.*

—II Corinthians 5:21

God wants us to be His children so badly that He was willing that
His son, Jesus, should come to earth as a man, live a sinless life, be
accused, suffer, and die a horrible death on the cross, in order that we,
by accepting Him for who He is and what He did, might be saved and
live forever in heaven.

*But God commendeth his love toward us, in that, while
we were yet sinners, Christ died for us.*

—Romans 5:8

*For God so loved the world, that he gave his only begotten
son, that whosoever believeth in him shall not perish, but
have everlasting life.*

—John 3:16

So that God, through His son Jesus, offers us eternal life

> *For the wages of sin is death; but the gift of God is eternal life through Jesus Christ our Lord.*
> —Romans 6:23

God is patient and wants all of us to accept Him, but just as He gave Adam and Eve a choice in the Garden, so He gives one to us.

> *The Lord is not slack concerning his promise, as some men count slackness; but is longsuffering to us-ward, not willing that any should perish, but that all should come to repentance.*
> —2 Peter 3:9

Yet we do not have a chance forever. If the Lord returns—or if we die without accepting Christ as our personal savior—the opportunity will have passed.

> *But the day of the Lord will come as a thief in the night; in the which the heavens shall pass away with a great noise, and the elements shall melt with fervent heat, the earth also and the works that are therein shall be burned up.*
> —2 Peter 3:10

The solution

> *That if thou shalt confess with thy mouth the Lord Jesus, and shalt believe in thine heart that God hath raised him from the dead, thou shalt be saved. For with the heart man believeth unto righteousness; and with the mouth confession is made unto salvation.*
> —Romans 10:9–10

Repent, confess, ask, and accept

When you decide that Jesus is who you want as your Lord and Savior, then pray.

Tell Him about your sin and ask forgiveness. Tell Him that you want Him to come into your heart and be your Lord and Savior. Ask Him to come in. And then the last step is vital: You must accept the gift He has given you, paid in full forgiveness and eternal life.

Knowing that you are going to heaven when you die makes all the difference. If you have more questions, or have made a decision to trust Jesus as your Savior and would like to share that wonderful news with me, please send an e-mail to kathyfae@gmail.com.

Appendix

Questions to Ask Your Doctor

When you are choosing a medical team, there several things to consider. Ask for referrals from friends who have been there. Who did they see? Did they have a good experience or not? Ask your personal physician. Ask a nurse. When you are meeting with the doctor you have chosen, ask the questions that follow.

Questions about the Medical Team

What is your personal experience with treating this form of cancer?

What are your qualifications?

What about a second opinion?

Should I go to a major cancer treatment center?

How will I contact you between appointments if I need something?

Do you have a Nurse Practitioner that will also work with me?

Information and Resources

Where can I get good information about my cancer and the treatment options?

Is there a social worker available and how can they be of help to me?

The Diagnosis

What do you suspect is wrong?

What kind of tests will I need to have?

Will I need surgery?

What kind of cancer do I have?

How aggressive is this form of cancer?

How progressed is my cancer?

Has it been staged? If so, what is the stage? And what exactly does that mean?

Has my cancer metastasized (gone anywhere else)?

If the cancer spreads, where does it normally go?

How will you monitor that?

What symptoms should I watch for?

The Treatment

What is the current recommended treatment for this type of cancer?

How many drugs are available?

What are the drug side effects I should expect?

Explain the difference between first and second line treatment drugs?

Will I need radiation treatments?

What are the risks?

Will I be asked to make choices about my treatment?

If so, what might they be?

Will I be sick?

Will I lose my hair?

Will I be able to continue working?

About the Author

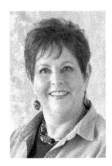

Kathy Manning Gronau lives in the Midwest. She is a retired RN/Counselor and has two sons and five grandchildren. In 2007 she lost her husband of forty-two years to colorectal cancer, and within a month was diagnosed with breast cancer. Now a survivor, she shares her experiences as a caregiver and patient. Her many insights from a nursing and counseling background will help you navigate the medical world and learn how to communicate with others, whether it be the patient or caregiver. You may communicate with Kathy at Kathymanninggronau@yahoo.com or on her website at www.eaticecreamforsupper.com

Additional Information from the Author

I sincerely hope that you've received value from *Eat Ice Cream for Supper: A Story of My Life with Cancer. A Guide for Your Journey.* By going through this process, I've learned more than I ever could have imagined. One of the most important things I realized is that when seeing a doctor for treatment or evaluation, asking the right questions, understanding and keeping track of their answers and how to act on them is vital. I've created the *Questions for the Doctor Notebook* for you to take to your doctors appointments so that you can ask the important questions and keep track of their answers. This tool is so important, that I want you to have it for FREE as my gift to you. Just go to http://kathymanninggronau.com/mygifttoyou to get your copy.

9 781614 488149